TRAINING THE WISDOM BODY

TRAINING THE WISDOM BODY

BUDDHIST YOGIC EXERCISE

Rose Taylor Goldfield

SHAMBHALA
BOSTON & LONDON
2013

Shambhala Publications, Inc.
Horticultural Hall
300 Massachusetts Avenue
Boston, Massachusetts 02115
www.shambhala.com

9 8 7 6 5 4 3 2 1

First Edition
Printed in the United States of America

♾ This edition is printed on acid-free paper that meets the
American National Standards Institute Z39.48 Standard.
♻ This book is printed on 30% postconsumer recycled paper.
For more information please visit www.shambhala.com.

Distributed in the United States by Random House, Inc.,
and in Canada by Random House of Canada Ltd

Designed by Gopa & Ted2, Inc.

Library of Congress Cataloging-in-Publication Data

Goldfield, Rose Taylor.
Training the wisdom body: Buddhist yogic exercise /
Rose Taylor Goldfield.—First edition
pages   cm
ISBN 978-1-61180-018-0 (pbk.)
1. Yoga. 2. Meditation—Buddhism. I. Title.
RA781.67.G65 2013
613.7'046—dc23
2012050840

Contents

ACKNOWLEDGMENTS

IT TOOK MANY people to transform this book from a vision to a reality, and I am grateful to everyone who helped in the process.

In particular, my heartfelt appreciation goes out to the following people who have been profound influences in my life and from whom I receive so much strength and support. To Bridget Taylor— my mother—for my life, for all she has taught me, and for introducing me to buddhadharma. We were together when we had the great good fortune to meet Khenpo Tsültrim Gyamtso Rinpoche (who would become my heart teacher) and his translator and secretary, Ari Goldfield (who would become my heart companion). To Ari—a wonderfully gifted teacher and my beloved husband—who holds me to a higher vision of myself and who brings learning, light, and laughter to our daily life together. I am so thankful to Khenpo Rinpoche for the opportunity to be his student; to work for him; to live with him; and to share the crazy, joyful, unsettling, dreamlike world that he inhabits, one that reverberates with song. I would also like to express my endless gratitude to Chögyam Trungpa Rinpoche for the extraordinary wealth of Dharma teachings that he has left to the world and to which I continually turn for succor, inspiration, and humor.

When I was studying Tibetan, it was hard to find people with the skill, time, and generosity to develop my studies further. I would like to express my sincere gratitude to those who helped me on that road—in particular, Lama Chönam, Jules Levinson, and Chryssoula Zerbini.

Now to the many people who worked specifically on this book, every one of whom I would be delighted to work with again (I feel so fortunate in being able to say that). Ari's help was invaluable throughout the entire process—planning, forming, and editing the book, as well as maintaining my sanity (or something resembling it). Heartfelt gratitude to Sara Bercholz for her skillful editing, which added a lot to the book, and for her friendship and support; also to the entire Shambhala Publications staff—it was wonderful to work with them again. I was far from looking forward to the photo shoot, expecting it to be rather excruciating, but it turned out to be a fun day under the kind professional care of expert photographer Claudine Gosset and the two lovely ladies who assisted me, Lisa Jacobs and Deb Wolfe. Lama Palden and Sukhasiddhi Foundation generously offered their space for the shoot. Many thanks to Chelsea Points for doing such a wonderful job on the illustrations and to Jeff Wigman for the excellent spine illustration. I am very grateful to two dear friends: Emily Bower, for her adept advice, and Annelies Smith, for her insightful reading of the draft manuscript. The snazzy outfit is courtesy of Beyond Yoga.

I would also like to add thanks to the following for their friendship and support: Stuart Lawson of Paragon Kickboxing Gym; Waylon Lewis of *Elephant Journal*; Lama Palden, John Roadhouse, Edward Taylor, and to all the truly delightful members of the Wisdom Sun Community.

INTRODUCTION

In 2007, I moved to Seattle with my teacher, Khenpo Tsültrim Gyamtso Rinpoche; his Tibetan attendant, Tsepak Dorje; and his translator and secretary for more than a decade, Ari Goldfield (who is now my husband). We stayed there for more than two years in semi-retreat. During that time, Khenpo Rinpoche first suggested that I write a book on the practice of *lujong.*

Lujong is a Tibetan compound word: *lu (lus)*[1] means "body," and *jong ('byong)* means "training" or "practice." It is a generic term like *exercise* in English and is used for many types of physical exercise that are practiced in Tibet. I call the practices described in this book Wisdom Body Lujong to differentiate them from other types of lujong. There are two ways to understand the term "wisdom body." First, the foundation for this movement practice is the wisdom teachings on reality, as explained in Part One of this book. This wisdom informs how we relate to our own bodies and these exercises. Second, as shown in Part Four, these exercises help us to connect with and explore the natural wisdom inherent in our living, breathing, feeling bodies.

During our period of retreat in Seattle, Khenpo Rinpoche encouraged me to further my lujong practice by incorporating what I had learned in my studies of other movement forms, including Indian, Chinese, and Japanese yogic systems and martial arts. At this time, I was also developing yogic dance practices under his guidance and studying the Newar tradition of sacred dance from the Kathmandu Valley. These profound practices have all greatly influenced my understanding and practice of meditational movement.

This book is my own interpretation of the teachings I received from my teacher and a synthesis of my personal history of movement practices. Khenpo Rinpoche authorized many teachers of lujong, and each of us has our own individual and unique take on this practice and teach from our personal background. This reflects Khenpo Rinpoche's own teaching path—after deep study and practice with his own teachers, he innovated in ways that have been extremely beneficial to those of us fortunate enough to study with him. Innovation and flexibility are hallmarks of his being and his teaching methods.

When Khenpo Rinpoche himself was traveling and teaching lujong, he would modify the exercises, teach them in different orders, and add exercises as students developed their practice. When asked where these exercises came from, he answered, "The Dharmadhatu," meaning "the expanse of genuine reality." While similar poses and exercises can be found in various Tibetan exercise systems, the way Khenpo Rinpoche teaches us to blend our minds with the profound view while moving our bodies is something at which he is particularly skilled and for which he is revered.

At first, this practice was restricted to a small group of his advanced students (and parts of the practice are still restricted to students who have reached a certain level of practice and experience). However, over the years, Khenpo Rinpoche began to teach the exercises more openly, believing that it was important and beneficial for everyone to learn how to combine meditation and exercise.

The intention of this book is to provide a thorough foundation for those who are new to Wisdom Body Lujong; to support continued practice for those who are already familiar with the exercises; and to help people engaged in any form of yogic exercise or meditation practice to deepen the potent fusion of meditation and physical movement.

Wisdom Body Lujong is practiced by people of all ages and all levels of physical ability. Because it is first and foremost a meditational exercise, the mental awareness you bring to the practice is the most important element—not the ability to contort your body into a particular pose. This series of exercises is quite simple to perform and can be varied in intensity depending on how your body feels when you begin each session. It is important to be aware of your body and to listen to it before, during, and after the session in order to avoid physical strain or injury and to awaken your body's inherent wisdom and compassion. All Buddhist practices are designed to increase wisdom and compassion, so it is essential to use both these elements in your body-based practices, particularly in how you relate to and care for your body in movement practice.

THE BENEFITS OF WISDOM BODY LUJONG

These days, we hear a lot about research in the areas of meditation and physical exercise and how beneficial they are for our physical, mental, and emotional well-being. By bringing our meditation and movement practice together, we receive all these benefits in a potent way.

In the classical teachings on meditation, there are two main obstacles to our practice: dullness and agitation. Meditational movement works as an antidote to both these obstacles. Moving the body diminishes the mind's dullness and keeps us alert and wakeful. With movement, we have a strong focal point of concentration, so the mind is less prone to agitation and distraction.

When we focus the mind in the present moment in time and the current location in space, we feel our awareness become embodied. Body and mind are synchronized. In our daily lives, we often find that mind and body become disconnected. This happens when mind disappears into replaying past events, projecting fantasies and fears onto the future, or fixating on some outer object of focus such as watching the little screens on our phones or computers. But when we focus the mind on the body, we bring body and mind back together.

Synchronizing body and mind in this way grounds us in present reality, helping us to feel stable, confident, and whole. We can relax into what is and not concern ourselves with what might be. In this space, we tune into the innate wisdom of our felt experience, which allows us to connect with our deep, internal guidance system. The real world opens up to us, and life becomes vivid, rich, even joyful, and definitely more workable.

The purpose of Wisdom Body Lujong is to work on our entire system, from the coarse aspects to the more subtle and profound. On the coarse physical level, the exercises enhance physical health and help us manage pain and illness. We also learn to connect with the body's innate energy. When we experience an energy dip in the middle of the day, we can tap into this resource instead of succumbing to the urge to reach for a sugary snack or caffeinated drink.

On a deeper level, we purify and release knotting within the energetic body that causes the internal winds to flow erratically and produces physical and emotional problems. When those knots loosen, we gain a greater sense of ease and equilibrium.

Ultimately, the highest purpose of this practice is to clarify our meditation experience, so that we can realize the true nature of reality—the true nature of our own being and everything with which we interact. We thereby can experience nondual wisdom-awareness, our complete connection to and inseparability from everything. This experience is open, spacious, and relaxed.

To attain such realization, we need to achieve pliancy of body and mind. As Khenpo Rinpoche once told me,

> In order to have a supple mind, you need a supple body.
> In order to have a supple body, you need a supple mind.
> So exert yourself in yogic exercise.[2]

It is through working with the body—an apparently solid entity made of flesh and blood—that we clear up our mistaken ideas about what the body is and realize its illusory nature. It is a completely fluid entity with no solid, fixed substance that we can grasp. It is in a state of continual change and movement. Similarly, as we meditate on the true nature of mind, we experience its natural fluidity and its ungraspable, continual dance of brilliant energy. The mind is said to be like the light of the sun and the moon, but the clouds of our belief that thoughts and feelings are fixed entities obscure that light. Once we overcome that mistaken belief, mind's luminous nature shines through. The inseparability of the illusory body and luminous mind is known as the *body of union*—complete buddhahood. This is the ultimate destination of our practice and, paradoxically, also its starting place, since this is the true nature of our being and our experience.

This Book

This book is divided into four parts. The first, "Foundations of Practice," includes an overview of the unique tradition of Buddhist yoga; presentations on the three foundational principles of renunciation, compassionate *bodhichitta*, and the profound view of reality; and an explanation of the three aspects—body, mind, and subtle body—that comprise our whole being.

Having established the foundation of practice in this way, the second part, "Seated Meditation Practice," explains how to work with the body and mind in seated meditation. The third part, "Extending Practice," explores ways we can further our practice by working with adversities such as fear, procrastination, and anxiety; by playing with vocalized practice using songs and syllables; and by looking at how to bring practice mind into daily life.

The final part, "Exercise Instructions," gives a complete explanation of the movement practices.

PART ONE
Foundations of Practice

I: BUDDHIST YOGA

Yogic consciousness . . . arises from meditation. . . .
When the net of concepts is cleared away,
Genuine reality vividly appears.[1]
—DHARMAKIRTI, SEVENTH-CENTURY INDIAN BUDDHIST MASTER

Although the disturbing emotions, the five poisons,[2]
　may agitate your mind,
Look at their true face, and let them be self-liberated.
Whatever thoughts of despair may arise in you,
Know their true nature and thereby gain courage.
When you know how to practice these points well,
You will be a relaxed yogini.[3]
—KHENPO TSÜLTRIM GYAMTSO RINPOCHE

THE TRADITION of Buddhist yoga is vast and wonderful. It is profound in the insights we can discover for our own and others' benefit, and it is rich in the variety of skillful methods we can use to put it into practice. This chapter presents the key points of this tradition[4] in a way that Buddhists and non-Buddhists alike will find helpful and applicable to their practices of yoga and meditation. These key points can be applied to a variety of activities beyond the exercises presented in this book, and in this way, they awaken us to the brilliance and richness present in each and every moment of our lives.

What makes Buddhist yoga so profound and transformational? To begin to answer this question, we will first examine the actual term so that we have a clear understanding of what we are talking about.

WHAT DOES "BUDDHIST YOGA" MEAN?

The words *Buddhist* and *yoga*—and by extension the names for adherents of yoga, male yogis and female yoginis—can have such a wide range of meanings and images that it is helpful to begin by looking precisely at the words' definitions.

Buddhist in Tibetan is *nangpa sangjeh pa* (*nang pa sangs rgyas pa*). *Nang pa* literally means "insider," but not in the sense of someone in a club or group separate from outsiders. Rather, it means "someone who looks inside"—someone who is not satisfied with the superficiality of life and wants to look deep into his or her experience and discover its true nature. It refers to people who want to look deep inside their own being to fully understand themselves.

Many of us spend much of our lives seeking satisfaction and happiness in the external world through our material possessions, family, work, social status, or relationships. Yet we often find that these things do not fulfill us in the ways we desire. Even when we do find some happiness in them, that happiness passes—it is not stable and lasting. We sense that it must be possible to feel more connected to our experiences, to know deeper levels of satisfaction and contentment, to open more fully with curiosity and playfulness to the magic and wonder of the world. Thus begins our Buddhist journey of discovering the true nature inside appearances and mind.

The word *nang* also connotes the sense of "home." We are not satisfied to hold our philosophical views at arm's length in a purely intellectual way. We want to bring them home, to have them transform the most personal and intimate aspects of our lives, even to transform our selves.

The second part of this term—*sangjeh* (*sangs rgyas*)—is the Tibetan word for "buddha," and each syllable is a word with its own meaning. *Sang* means "awaken," or to awaken from our ignorance, which makes us suffer in a variety of ways because we are not in harmony with reality. Because our mistaken thinking does not correspond with the way things are, friction is created between the two. In consequence, we experience all kinds of suffering: anxiety, stress, discomfort, and disconnect. When we awaken from this sleep of ignorance, we reconnect with the wisdom that is in complete harmony with reality; our journey through life becomes smoother.

This reality—meaning the reality of our own mind and all the phenomena it perceives—is awareness. Awareness transcends conceptual labels and expressions, and it even transcends the duality between the outer objects we perceive and our inner consciousnesses that perceive them. It has the qualities of openness, spaciousness, and relaxation, and it is available to us even in our most troubling experiences. It is what enables us to be truly at peace and in harmony.

Another meaning of *sang* is "to purify." What we purify or eliminate are all our habitual, automatic patterns of thinking and behaving that shut down the vivid reality of present experience. We eliminate them because they cause us to suffer, and that, in turn, causes us to increase the suffering of those around us; it is hard to be there for others, to be kind, generous, and thoughtful, when we are ensnared in our own suffering. The whole of the Buddhist path is about giving up behavior that does not serve ourselves or others and about adopting behavior that supports finding true happiness for all.

The next syllable refers to the qualities that increase. *Jeh* means "expand," referring to how the qualities of enlightenment such as clarity, equanimity, love, compassion, and happiness all grow from having awakened into wisdom. In fact, these qualities are inherent within mind's true nature, and through training in Buddhist yoga, our ability to actualize them grows and grows. Thus, no matter what religious, spiritual, or philosophical tradition we may follow (or not), we act in harmony with Buddhist principles when we look beneath the surface of appearances, thoughts, and emotions into their true nature; when we train in awakening from ignorance into wisdom that realizes this true nature; and when we practice engendering compassion and the other qualities of enlightenment.

Yoga in Tibetan is *naljor* (*rnal 'byor*), meaning "to join (*jor*) with naturalness (*nal ma*), the true nature of reality." Yoga, therefore, is any and all of the practices by which we join with naturalness and achieve our awakening into wisdom and compassion. Yogis and yoginis are not distinguished by wearing special clothes, eating certain foods, or sitting in particular postures; anyone dedicated to practicing on the path of joining with naturalness is a yogi or yogini. As the great Tibetan yogi Milarepa[5] explained, "In my tradition, if you sincerely want to practice the Dharma, you do not have to change your name. Since you can reach buddhahood with a full head of hair, you do not have to cut it off or change your clothes."[6]

The transformation we aspire to is not merely a superficial aesthetic one but something that goes to the heart of our experience. Such a transformation cannot be displayed in coarse forms, such as our manner of dress or hairstyle, but can only truly be known in our hearts; this is called self-awareness. We each know our own experience intimately; no one else can truly know it. It is inexpressible because it is a felt experience beyond conceptual terms.

How Do We Join with Naturalness?

To join with the naturalness of the outer material world, we ascertain the true nature of matter and rest within it. To join with the naturalness of mind, we ascertain the true nature of mind and rest within it. The body is the perfect focus for doing both of these kinds of yoga, because as Milarepa taught, the body is the border region where mind and matter meet. The body is made of what is commonly considered matter, yet that matter is suffused with mental sensation and feeling—in other words, mind. Body and mind are interdependent: changes in the body affect the mind, and the mind's perceptions and feelings bring about physical changes. By penetrating to the true nature of the body, we discover the true nature of mind, and by ascertaining mind's true nature, we discover the true nature of the body. Ultimately, our practice of Buddhist yoga reveals to us that the difference between body and mind is merely a conceptual one, and in reality—nondual, inexpressible awareness—body and mind are inseparable.

This is why it is skillful to employ both body and mind on the path to enlightenment. If we were to focus too heavily on one or the other, our practice would be out of balance. The key, therefore, is to give appropriate attention to each and to train in their interrelationship by involving mind when we work with body and involving body when we work with mind. Then our practice is balanced and whole, and we make good use of all available resources on our journey. We will begin to see how to do this in the following chapters on the three qualities of mind we develop to give our yoga practice its soundest possible foundation.

2: RENUNCIATION

THE FIRST PRINCIPLE we work with in Buddhist yoga is renunciation, which can be a challenging idea. It may sound like we are being taught to renounce the people we love, the activities we enjoy, our work—in short, to give up life as we have lived it. But this is not the case. Since Buddhism focuses on working with ourselves from the inside out rather than the outside in, its teachings do not command us to do anything. Instead, they invite us to investigate things for ourselves and come to our own conclusions as to how to proceed. That is the only way we will be stable and confident in our actions.

In the case of renunciation, what we are invited to explore is how happiness and suffering operate. Our usual tendency is to look for happiness outside ourselves. We think that by manipulating our environment and the objects in it—by accumulating the material possessions and resources we desire, being treated in a particular way by others, perfecting our physical bodies, and so forth—we can make our internal experience one of contentment and happiness.

But the harder and faster we chase these butterflies of ephemeral, external happiness, the further we remove ourselves from the true and stable source of happiness within our own heart and mind.

Thus, what we renounce, or let go of, is our mistaken expectation that manipulating the world will bring us happiness. However, it is certainly true that our external circumstances and relationships affect our well-being and peace of mind, so we do need to pay attention to them. Rejecting the outer world and devaluing our relationship with it would be going too far to the other extreme.

And there is nothing wrong with enjoying the pleasures of life like our morning tea, our friends, the beauty of nature, and our favorite chocolate. It is simply that by developing qualities within ourselves and working on our internal sense of contentment and joy, we learn to be with ourselves as we are, with other people as they are, and with the world as it is, without struggle. So if we have these pleasurable things, we enjoy them in a spacious and relaxed way; if we do not have them, we are less disturbed. We have a greater sense of equanimity and peace.

The Tibetan word for renunciation, *ngayjung* (*nges 'byung*), has the connotation of "emergence." The Tibetan master Chögyam Trungpa Rinpoche described the cocoon that we construct for ourselves from our mistaken beliefs and habitual patterns. It may be a little claustrophobic, smelly, and dark in our cocoon, but at least it is familiar; we have a cowardly belief that the devil we know is better than something unknown.

Renunciation asks us to be courageous and emerge from our cocoons into the vast expanse of reality. Initially, we may feel vulnerable, fearful, or nostalgic for our cocoon, but in the long term, we find a genuine and vivid world of deep, sincere engagement. We wake up to reality and see things simply as they are. We become fully, openly, and directly immersed in life. Instead of living our lives from the outside in—focusing on outer achievements rather than inner fulfillment, on how our physical body looks rather than how it feels, on the quantity of our friendships rather than their quality—we learn to live from the inside out. We focus on our core feelings, intuition, and integrity, and we give our hearts a more prominent role in guiding our actions in the world.

CORRECTING A BASIC MISTAKE

We can more easily live in the way just described if we correct a basic mistake in the way we think about things—that they are existent, fixed, permanent, and solid. We do this with ourselves, our bodies, our feelings, our friends, our jobs, everything (even our spiritual path), and when we do, we exaggerate each thing's importance and our relationship with it becomes heavy. For example, we view the body as permanent, and we want it to always be healthy, so we become distressed by any sign of weakness or sickness. We view our friends and family as fixed entities, and we want them to always love us and treat us well, exposing us to constant disappointment. Most of all, we think that the mind is a real entity, and we want it to be happy and free of any agitation, worry, or anguish. We forget the truth of the poet Rainer Maria Rilke's aphorism "No feeling is final." When we experience a feeling, especially a difficult one, it seems like the most important thing in the world. This makes us feel stuck and even hopeless. We forget that we have had other feelings before, and in the future, a whole variety of new feelings will arise.

When we ignore the reality of impermanence, fluidity, and change in all these areas, we approach life with the belief that we should be able to organize everything in life so that it suits us and feels comfortable. We place this completely unrealistic expectation on ourselves and the world, and then we suffer from our lack of control over things and how they change in ways that we do not like. We suffer from physical aging and sickness, from conflict in our relationships, from uncertainty and downturns in our work and livelihood. We resist the impermanent nature of things—the way in which life is always changing and unpredictable. We struggle to fix and solidify our world rather than relaxing and letting ourselves flow with its transitions and cyclical phases.

The Buddhist teachings invite us to look at our lives and ask, "Has my attempt to solidify my world worked? Has believing in the true existence of my body, mind, friends, family, and work ever brought me lasting happiness? Or has it just made me vulnerable to suffering?" If through this examination, we become certain that there is no happiness to be found in clinging to things as truly existent, then that is authentic renunciation. It does not mean that we have to disregard or abandon our physical well-being, material possessions, or friends; it only means we stop clinging to them—particularly as being solid entities, which they are not. As the great Indian master Tilopa sang to his disciple, Naropa,

> Appearances do not bind you, your clinging binds you.
> So cut through your clinging, my son Naropa.[1]

When we cut through our clinging and interact with our bodies, people, and other things in our lives, our relationships with them are more relaxed, allowing us to feel more at ease. This does not mean, however, that we are no longer able to differentiate between pleasure and pain or that we do not experience emotions, such as deep sadness at the loss of a loved one. It means that we no longer struggle with our experiences of suffering. We know they are not solid and fixed, that their nature is to change. Then the difficult feelings we experience are softer and more manageable; we experience them as part of the tapestry of life rather than as solid, overwhelming, and unworkable forces. Living in this way, we allow emotions to remain fluid, which releases their pure, underlying energy—the fuel for our journey of joining with naturalness.

3: COMPASSIONATE BODHICHITTA

THE SECOND QUALITY cultivated by practitioners of Buddhist yoga is *bodhichitta* ("the awakening mind"), the motivation to attain buddhahood for the benefit of all sentient beings. By fully awakening to the reality of ourselves and our world, we are able to help others reach the same realization, which brings freedom from confused suffering and genuine happiness. The great masters have taught that bodhichitta is the most positive and powerful motivation we can have for our practice. As the Indian teacher Shantideva (seventh–eighth century) proclaimed,

> If with kindly generosity
> One merely has the wish to soothe
> The aching heads of other beings,
> Such merit knows no bounds.
> No need to speak, then, of the wish
> To drive away the endless pain
> Of each and every living being,
> Bringing them unbounded excellence.[1]

'awakened mind'

What ignites our bodhichitta is compassion, the wish that sentient beings will be free from suffering. Compassion keeps our practice free of small-minded purpose, gives it great energy, and keeps our mind open and spacious. And compassion is accessible to everyone, because it is inherent in mind's true nature. Remembering that compassion is innate is important, because it gives us confidence in our ability to be kind and caring. We simply need to help this natural ability manifest.

The main way to develop compassion is to generate good feelings toward others. First, bring to mind someone of whom you are very fond and recall how you enjoy being with that person and the times when he or she has helped you. As you contemplate this, feel the warmth and joy that it brings to your heart. Feel yourself and the other person bathed in these warm, connected, and loving feelings.

Then expand that natural friendliness toward those for whom you have no particular feelings. You can think about all the people with whom you interact on a regular basis but whom you do not consider either friends or enemies: the bus driver who takes you to work each day, your local grocery store cashiers, people you regularly pass as you walk your dog.

To help in this endeavor, recall the humanity—the beingness—we all share. All sentient beings have the desire to be happy, yet we all regularly experience various kinds of suffering: from daily frustrations and stress due to problems at work, traffic jams, and long lines when we are in a hurry to more severe difficulties such as relationship breakups, the loss of a job, or the death of a loved one. All of us go through these experiences, and all of us constantly face the truth of impermanence and our own impending death. The more we are aware of this, the easier it is to extend warmth to others.

When you have some practice with these levels of compassion, try extending the warmth and friendliness even further—to people you find difficult and whom you tend to view in a negative way or those for whom you feel hatred or anger. This can be extremely challenging. But the more you understand that everyone is subject to the first of Buddhism's Four Noble Truths (the truth of suffering), the greater your ability to extend your compassion to unsympathetic people. From a psychological perspective, it is often true that those who inflict the most suffering have themselves been the victims of physical and mental abuse. So they are often deeply in need of understanding and compassion. In this practice, the focus is simply to work on your own judgment of and inability to look kindly on these people. At this stage, you do not necessarily directly engage these people. The first step is to work with your own mind by looking to see what blocks your compassion and what is possible in terms of dissolving these blockages.

The compassion of Buddhist yoga is known as "great compassion," or *nyingjay chenpo* (*snying rje chen po*), because its vast scope includes friends and enemies alike. Ordinary compassion is what we feel for those of whom we are fond and those we consider worthy of compassion, such as the victims of aggression. It is not for our enemies or people we dislike, such as the perpetrators of aggressive acts, whom we feel are unworthy of compassion. Buddhist yoga invites us to begin to consider friends and enemies, victims and aggressors, in a more equal way. To the extent that people are lost in mistaken beliefs and confusion, everyone suffers and is worthy of compassion. And everyone has within them the buddhanature, the pure true nature of mind and heart. So all beings—friends, enemies, victims, and aggressors—are equally worthy of compassion.

The following verse, commonly recited in Tibetan Buddhism, is an excellent way to focus the mind to arouse these qualities of love and compassion for all beings:

> May all beings have happiness and the causes of happiness,
> May they be free from suffering and the causes of suffering,
> May they always have genuine happiness that is
> untarnished by suffering,
> And may they reside in great equanimity, free of attachment
> and anger toward anyone near or far.[2]

The term "all beings" is abstract. It is not so hard to be compassionate with abstract beings, but it can be very difficult with real beings of flesh and blood with whom we have direct relationships! So if you choose to work with this verse, I encourage you to make the beings real for you; think of specific people in specific situations.

Although relationships with some people are often messy, and we may feel that it is easier not to have to deal with them, we also have good reason to be grateful to them. It is in relation to others that we are able to develop our own good qualities of love, compassion, generosity, and patience. In fact, these qualities only arise in relationship with others. And it is in these relationships that we test the strength of these qualities within ourselves and discover where we get stuck and have further work to do.

Also, the more we learn about the nature of reality, the more our compassion awakens and expands. We discover that in genuine reality—nondual and luminous awareness—there is no difference between me and you, between self and other; there is no difference between the true nature of one being's mind and that of another. The mind of all beings is basically good. Whatever faults we and other sentient beings may appear to have, they are all temporary. As practitioners of Buddhist yoga, we develop compassion for all beings that is grounded in our awareness of our inherent equality with others and their equality with us.

WORKING WITH COMPASSIONATE BODHICHITTA

Sometimes the subtlety of the teachings on compassionate bodhichitta gets lost in our attempt to apply these teachings to our own lives. Compassionate bodhichitta is not the same as people-pleasing. These teachings are not instructions to disavow our own needs while attempting to fulfill the arbitrary desires of those around us.

Genuine compassion is imbued with great wisdom that considers the full picture in order to judge what action is most beneficial in a given circumstance. Sometimes this may not be the action that will make us most popular, but genuine compassion is not about winning a popularity contest—it does what is most beneficial for all concerned. For example, parents understand that in raising their children, it is important not to simply indulge them but to provide boundaries and guidance that endow them with skills to create a good life for themselves.

While engaging in compassionate activity, it is important to remember the free will of those with whom we work. It is not within our power to completely transform someone else's life. Even the Buddha could only show us the way to deep personal transformation; it is up to us to take those steps ourselves. While it is within our power to help others, there is no way to completely satisfy and please people. Even Milarepa admitted, "Trying to please others is endless."[3] For every desire we meet for someone else, another will arise to replace it. Just as it does not serve us to indulge our own desires, it is not helpful to try to satisfy all those of another person. As Trungpa Rinpoche put it,

> We cannot just be "love-and-light" bodhisattvas. If we do not work intelligently with sentient beings, quite possibly our help will become addictive rather than beneficial. People will become addicted to our help in the same way they become addicted to sleeping pills. By trying to get more and more help they will become weaker and weaker.[4]

Just like good parents, what we really want to encourage in others is internal strength, not dependency. To further our altruistic activity, we need to keep increasing our wisdom so we know what is truly beneficial in any given situation. One way to do this is to look deeply into our own mind and heart and examine our own motivations. At the core of our compulsive self-sacrificing for others we sometimes find a deep sense of worthlessness or a belief that the only way that we will be safe or loved is to negate our own needs and provide for the needs of others. The more we illuminate our own compulsions and habits, the further we erode our filters of mistaken beliefs. Not only does this bring us great relief, but it also gives us much more clarity in our compassionate activity and provides a wonderful example to others.

It is also worth remembering that the line from the previous verse—"May all beings have happiness and the causes of happiness"—applies to us too. We are worthy of the same level of care that we show others. As the Buddha taught in the sutra called *The King of Meditative States,*

> All wandering beings are completely pervaded by the
>   enlightened essence,
> All wandering beings, without exception, are precisely
>   buddha,
> Therefore, all sentient beings are worthy.[5]

In this modern era of globalization, we see how interconnected and interdependent we all are in immediate and obvious ways. For us to be truly happy as individuals, all of society and all forms of sentient beings need to be respected and cared for. So when cultivating compassion, rather than swapping our focus from ourselves to others, we extend our focus to include all other beings without excluding ourselves in the process.

THE POWER OF GENTLENESS

Compassionate intention also gives us great strength—sometimes, literal physical strength. You have probably heard stories like that of Angela Cavallo, who in 1982 was able to lift the side of a car beneath which her son was trapped and hold it for approximately five minutes while others pulled the boy to safety. She probably could not have done that in normal circumstances, but when we really connect with the desire to help another person, something that seemed impossible may become possible. As the third Jamgon Kongtrul Rinpoche taught, "There is nothing as strong as true gentleness, and there is nothing as gentle as true strength."

You can experiment with developing the power of gentleness while practicing movement meditation. For example, in one yoga class I took, after performing one pose, we were instructed to repeat the posture having first aroused a mind of compassion toward someone we wished to benefit. I thought of my mother, how much I appreciate our relationship, and my desire to alleviate any suffering she might have. Then I held the posture and dedicated it to her. By using this simple technique, I was able to hold the pose longer and with more precision and energy. You can try similar experiments to see how mind's power increases when you harness it to a positive, altruistic end.

In Buddhist yoga, we are taught to arouse the mind of bodhichitta before every practice. This infuses our whole practice with the power of compassion. At the end of every practice, we dedicate its positive results to others. Dedicating the merit of our practice is classically compared to pouring a glass of water into a great ocean. The fruits of our individual efforts may seem small, but when dedicated to others, they join with a vast ocean of positive, altruistic energy.

The act of giving away our merit rather than hoping for some return for ourselves creates the energy of openness and generosity. It challenges our normal energetic pattern of attempting to hold on to good things for ourselves. And as we increase our energy of openness and kindness, we make a positive impact on our world.

4: Joining with Naturalness through the Profound View of True Reality

THE THIRD QUALITY of mind that Buddhist yogis and yoginis need is the view of the profound true nature of reality—nondual awareness. This is the awareness we find beyond our mistaken constructs of reality, the most basic of which is the belief that "I" (as the perceiving subject) and all that is "other" than me (all the objects that I perceive) are separate from each other.

A sign that we are starting to experience nondual awareness comes in our meditation practice, when we feel spacious, relaxed, and clear; when it feels like rigidity is beginning to dissolve; and when we feel less of a distance between ourselves and our world. The more this happens, the more our feelings of aloneness and other disturbing emotions weaken. We are joining with naturalness. The great yogis and yoginis describe this experience in beautiful ways, with words like *relaxed, luminous, blissful,* and *immutable.* The Indian yogini Niguma sang:

> What throws you down into samsara's deep ocean
> Are these thoughts of attachment and anger.
> But realize they don't truly exist,
> And all is an island of gold![1]

The Lord of Yogis, Milarepa, in his song "Eighteen Kinds of Yogic Joy," sang,

The bliss is good in the expanse of the confidence of
strength of mind.
What develops on its own by its own force feels extremely
good.[2]

And in "Ten Things It's Like," he sang,

When your conduct is free of all adopting and all rejecting
The mind just settles down in a space that's action-free
And this mind that settles down in a space that's action-free
Is like the body and the mind and roar of a lion in his prime.

Bright appearance, bright emptiness, and wisdom bright
Are like the blazing sun when it's shining in a cloud-free
sky.[3]

Khenpo Tsültrim Gyamtso Rinpoche sang,

Look nakedly at these forms that are like rainbows,
appearance-emptiness,
Listen intently to these sounds that are like echoes,
sound-emptiness,
Look straight at the essence of mind—clarity-emptiness,
inexpressible,
And fixation-free, at ease in your own nature, let go and
relax. Ahh, ahh, ahh.[4]

STAGE ONE OF JOINING WITH NATURALNESS: THE SELFLESSNESS OF BODY AND MIND

To help us realize this profound true nature, the Buddha taught how
to gain certainty in it and meditate in stages.[5] These stages help us
to see the mistakes present in the way we ordinarily think about

things and how to rectify those mistakes with clearer understanding and experience. Along the way, our anxiety, confusion, and suffering diminish, and the spaciousness, clarity, and happiness that are naturally present within our minds emerge.

The following is a very brief presentation of these topics. They are profound teachings, and it takes a long time to realize their subtlety and true meaning and then to incorporate that into our lives. If your curiosity is aroused and you have many questions, that is great! There are many ways to continue exploring these themes.[6]

The first stage is to realize the selflessness of the individual—meaning that in body and mind, there is no solidly existent, fixed entity of "self." All of our suffering comes from thoughts such as, "I'm angry," "I'm sick," "I'm hurt," and "I'm in pain." But all of these thoughts are predicated on the belief that there really is an "I" and a "me." It is helpful to understand that the self that appears in our thoughts is like a dream, an illusion. This is the truth of selflessness.

We gain certainty in selflessness through the analysis of our own body and mind. Before analyzing, we may think we have one self that has a continuous existence from birth to death. But we must think about where in body and mind this single, continuously existing self is to be found.

At times, we may strongly identify with one part of the body; for example, when we have stomach pain and think, "I'm sick," because that part of the body is sick. But the body is not one thing; it is actually a multiplicity of parts. These parts are continually changing—constantly arising and dissolving, with new components replacing the old. Could any of this multitude of impermanent parts really be "me"?

When we investigate mind, we find no fixed or solid self. We have strong thoughts and emotional experiences with which we identify, like when we think, "I'm afraid," or "I'm upset." But we had experiences like that last year too, and they were replaced by other experiences, which were then replaced by yet other thoughts and emotions. Could any of these constantly changing thoughts and emotions really be "me"?

In our analysis, we find that the self only exists as a conceptual fixation. Our thoughts are prone to fixate on one part of the body or one event in the mind and think, "That's me." But do we feel good when we think like that? Usually, the stronger our thought of "me," the more tension and pain we feel. In contrast, the more we can join with selflessness, the more relaxed, clear, and happy we are. We realize that who we are is not defined by our successes or failures. We feel less need to grasp success and fear failure, and our experience becomes easier. The feelings of separation and loneliness that accompany ego-clinging begin to dissolve, which feels wonderful. As the Tibetan yogi Kalu Rinpoche taught,

> If you wake up to . . . reality,
> You will know that you are nothing,
> And being nothing, you are everything.[7]

We can still use the terms *I, me,* and *mine,* just as the Buddha did, because they are useful in helping us communicate, but when we do, we remain aware of the truth that this is only an illusory self, not a fixed and solid entity.

STAGE TWO OF JOINING WITH NATURALNESS: THE EMPTINESS OF BODY AND MIND

Body and mind are not only of the nature of selflessness, they are also of the nature of emptiness. *Emptiness*—which the Buddha taught to be the true nature of all phenomena—means that whatever phenomenon appears to our senses or thoughts, it does not truly exist. It is a mere appearance, like that in a dream or an illusion, and its true nature is beyond duality, beyond concept and expression.

Emptiness is too profound for most of us to be able to grasp immediately. However, if we approach it in a step-by-step way, we can understand it, gain certainty in it, and experience it in the same way that great yogis and yoginis do.

Let us begin this gradual approach into emptiness by analyzing the body. We have a conceptual idea of it, but when we actually try to find the body, we cannot, because "body" is just a label, a name given to a collection of smaller parts. If you try to identify your body by pointing to it, you cannot do so. When you point, your finger may touch your head, chest, arm, or leg, but it never identifies an entity called "body." The same is true when you try to point to your arm—you can point to the upper arm, lower arm, or hand, but "arm" is also just a name given to a collection of smaller parts. This is true for everything down to the subtle particles that comprise the body; each part is merely a name given to a collection of smaller parts, and those parts themselves are just collections of smaller parts. Therefore, the body is not actually made of any substance that can be found through analysis. The body is empty of matter, so its true nature is emptiness, and its appearance is like a rainbow or a body of pure light. As Milarepa sang,

> My body is appearance-emptiness, like a rainbow in
>   the sky.
> It cannot be identified, so my attachment to it has
>   dissolved.[8]

Mind's nature is also emptiness, because in essence, it is inexpressible and inconceivable. For example, if you eat a piece of fine chocolate, you have a mental experience that you cannot convey in words. You may describe it as sweet or delicious, but if you are asked, "What is sweet like? What is delicious like?" you quickly run out of words that can express your experience. The same is true for even the strongest emotions. If you have the feeling "I'm angry," but then you go past the label "anger" into the experience itself, you discover that no words can actually explain it.

This is true for happiness, sadness, calm, worry, pleasure, and pain—all the labels we superimpose on mind cannot actually describe mind's inexpressible nature. When we transcend those labels and rest in that inexpressible nature of mind, we experience the Dharmakaya—the enlightened mind of the Buddha that is our own mind's true nature—and the clarity, bliss, and emptiness that are inseparable from it. As Milarepa sang,

> All thoughts are free in being Dharmakaya,
> It's awareness, clarity, and bliss,
> So to meditate, rest uncontrived.[9]

BODY AND MIND'S ULTIMATE NATURE

The ultimate naturalness of body and mind is that they are inseparable. As the Indian yogi Dombe Heruka sang,

> Body and mind—nonduality,
> Spacious and relaxed transparency.[10]

The body, free of self, free of particles of matter, is the dance and play of mind's native luminosity. The experience of joining with this naturalness is like dancing in a dream when you know you are dreaming. Dualistic thoughts dissolve, and nondual awareness—luminous and blissful—manifests. This is the fruition of Buddhist yoga.

5: Body, Mind, and Subtle Body

As we discovered in the preceding chapters, the ultimate nature of the physical body and mind is the dance and play of wisdom-awareness. This is also true of the third aspect of our experience, which is called the *subtle body*. By understanding these three aspects, we can access them experientially and, from there, unfold our experience into our inherent wisdom-awareness.

The Physical Body

The physical body is the visible, tangible one that we can see at work in our lives. As we learned in chapter 4, it is not truly made of particles of matter but is rather a mere appearance of solidified energy that we refer to as having material substance. If this physical body is dissected, we find substances such as bone, muscle, fascia, and blood. It is our more obvious or coarse way of engaging with the world, which can be easily disassembled and examined. But a body without mind is an insensible mass; of this we can have no experience.

Much of our sense of duality is wrapped up in our experience of the body. For example, we feel that there is a definite boundary within which we have the power to compel movement and experience sensation, and outside of which we have no control. This leads us to conclude that part of the fabric of our experiential universe is "me" and "mine" while the other part of it is "other."

Through the precise logical reasonings of Buddhist yoga, we find that these distinctions are actually mistaken concepts. We find no such solid boundaries—our physical being is continually changing and mingling with the external environment. We take in foods, fluids, and oxygen and exchange them for bodily waste products. Even though we think of the body as a discrete entity, it is made of cells that are being shed moment to moment. So when do those external things we take in become "me"? And when we lose or excrete some material from the body, when does it change from "me" to "other"?

THE MIND

The mind is a subtler energetic entity. We know we experience something we can call *mind*, but we cannot pinpoint where it resides. In the West, we think our mind is somehow related to the material substance of our brain. In Tibet, the mind is thought to reside at the heart center. Neither point of view can ultimately be proved valid, because mind cannot be examined in the way that material substance can.

Scientists may posit that in brain imaging they can see certain points of the brain light up during a particular experience, but that does not prove a locus for mind. For example, the lighted areas may lead a scientist to conclude that you are feeling happy. But if you are actually feeling sad, confused, or anxious, is the scientist's instrument correct, or are you?

Mind is invisible, beyond the world of physical matter, beyond that which the senses can perceive. At the same time, it is mind that knows the perceptions of the five types of sense objects—sights, sounds, smells, tastes, and physical sensations. Mind without body would have no way to perceive the world and would remain in a state of isolation. So physical matter and mind are intricately connected.

THE SUBTLE BODY

The subtle body is another aspect of our whole being; it is our felt experience that lies somewhere between the physical body and the mind. We connect with the subtle body when we open to feelings, sensations, and patterns of energy in the physical body.

Try just feeling into your heart area; simply observe whatever sensation you find there. As you feel into it, see if the sensation changes in any way. Is the sensation heavy or light? Does it move, or does it seem stuck and solid? Is there a color, pattern, or image associated with this sensation? Are there internal areas that feel pulled in a particular direction or twisted in some way? What is your felt internal landscape? If you do not feel anything, feel into that nothingness—open to the experience of numbness, dullness, or deadened sensation. That, too, is a felt experience.

As we open to our felt sensations, we often find that they do not reflect the measurable physical body. Some areas feel as tiny and sharp as a pinpoint, while other areas feel like deep valleys or mountaintops. We feel patterns twisting and pulled in ways that do not necessarily reflect the tissues or position of the physical body. These are all experiences of the energetic subtle body.

In the Tibetan system, the subtle body is spoken of in terms of *tsa* (*rtsa*), *lung* (*rlung*), and *tiglay* (*thig le*)—the energy channels, inner winds, and energy beads or drops. There are many elaborate diagrams of the different channels and energy centers, and although some basic points (such as the central channel running from the pelvic floor up to the crown of the head, or "third eye") are universal, others (such as the number and colors of the energy centers located along the central channel) can vary a lot. So the subtle body can be pictured in different ways, depending on what practice we are doing. It is helpful to let go of conceptually fixating on what we think the subtle body should look like and contorting our experience to fit this external structure. Let us instead feel into our own individual experience of the subtle body, as did the yogis and yoginis who composed these descriptions.

THE THREEFOLD BEING IN MOVEMENT

As we practice the lujong exercises, we always engage all three aspects of our being. Our physical body is engaged in the movement, but the mind is not thinking of this body as a mass of material matter. Rather the mind keeps flashing on the true essence of the body: appearance-emptiness, like a dream body, a body of light, a rainbow in the sky, or a magical emanation. At times we use specific aspects of subtle body visualization (explained in the exercise instructions), but in general, we connect with the subtle body by meditating on the felt experience of the physical body and the sensations that arise for us, and by expanding into the sensation of how it feels to move—not as a solid, heavy body, but as a feeling body of light.

PART TWO

Seated Meditation Practice

6: CALM-ABIDING MEDITATION

NOW THAT WE know the foundational view of Buddhist yoga, we can bring this view into practice. To practice meditational movement, it is best to have experience in seated meditation, which we will explore in this section.

The Tibetan name for the basic foundational meditation technique is *shinnay* (*zhi gnas*), which means "calm-abiding." Through meditation, we learn to work with our thoughts. An untrained mind roams wildly from one thought to the next; there is little space, and the thinking process can feel out of control. Thoughts we do not want keep popping up and forcing themselves on us. Things we need to focus on keep eluding us. This leads to many difficulties. By training the mind, we gain more control over its activity and abide with more calmness.

The Buddhist tradition teaches that what binds us in states of suffering and dissatisfaction is actually nothing other than our own mind. Often we think that external circumstances create our suffering: we do not get what we want; we get what we do not want; material resources or possessions are somehow unsatisfactory; people do not behave as we wish. The list of external sources for dissatisfaction and unhappiness is endless. As discussed in chapter 2, Buddhism invites us to seek happiness from within. We are encouraged to stop relying on external circumstances for contentment, because they are fundamentally unreliable—even if somehow the world were ideally arranged for our happiness, experience shows that this can never last. At the very least, we will be separated from this happiness by death. What can provide lasting happiness are our own mind and heart.

Life can be as unpredictable as the weather—the sky can be calm and bright for many days, and then without warning, a storm strikes, throwing our lives into disarray. Or we wake up to an overcast day, expecting little from it, and by midmorning, the clouds part and glorious sunshine envelops us. We never know quite what is going to happen. But when we prepare ourselves by developing our internal resources, we can adapt to all kinds of weather.

It is common to long for a perfect lover, an ideal parent, some godlike being who—if we can just persuade him or her with our love, devotion, and compliance—will take away our pain and fulfill our desires. However, if this approach has failed us so far, it may be time to take on the task ourselves. This may sound disappointing initially, but it is also greatly empowering. Freeing ourselves from our discomfort and finding a sense of peace and joy is completely within our own abilities. But it does require commitment and energy to do the work it takes. We need to sit down and work with our own heart and feelings.

In choosing to work with mind and heart, we make a gesture of supreme friendliness toward ourselves. It is the best act of self-care. Each of us becomes a fully adult human being by taking responsibility for our lives and our well-being. In the beginning, we may feel that we have to draw into ourselves a little for this undertaking; however, we eventually realize that this is a gesture of friendliness not only to ourselves but also to others. If we all took complete responsibility for ourselves, it would have a powerful impact on the world.

This self-reliance does not negate our interdependence and our need for care and love from others. Actually, it is a strong person who knows he or she needs help and can ask for it. Equally, when we take care of ourselves, we find we are in a much better place to help those around us when they need it. By learning to be alone with our own mind, we learn how to be in relationship. If we have not come to terms with our own confusion, emotions, and habitual patterns, these unresolved issues will affect our interactions with others.

Take care of your shit.

The good news is that the more we get to know our own mind in meditation practice, the more at ease we become with ourselves. We find we can actually be with difficult states of mind without having to try to avoid them through entertainment, alcohol, social-izing, shopping, eating, or whatever method we use to numb our experience. It is not that we no longer have difficult states of mind; it is that through meditation we develop a ground that makes them workable.

CONCEPTUAL MIND AND NONCONCEPTUAL EXPERIENCE

We can make our mind workable by refining our understanding of mind's conceptual and nonconceptual modes of experience and learning how to work with them effectively. The mode of conceptu-ality, or thoughts, is to proliferate. This is problematic, because the more we follow conceptual mind, the more our experience speeds up. We feel a sense of compulsion, like a hamster running on an exercise wheel—we keep running, the wheel turns faster, and we do not know how to slow down, let alone get off. Not only does this feel uncomfortable and exhausting, but it also greatly limits our experience.

We feel the negative impact of this on the internal winds of our subtle body. The mind rides on the internal winds, and conversely, the winds also follow the mind's placement of attention. So if we focus our attention in the lower belly, as we will learn to do in part 3 of this book, then the internal winds will be directed there. But when our attention is with conceptual mind, the focus is in our head, so the internal winds rise up and gather in the upper body, often in the chest, shoulders, neck, and head. This is why we often accumulate tension in those areas when we work on tasks that require a lot of thought or when we use a computer. If this happens repeatedly and is not corrected, the result is a *wind disorder*, whose symptoms are feelings of tension, anxiety, stress, and depression.

In contrast, our nonconceptual awareness is our direct perception of sense experience via the physical body. All that we experience through the physical senses is grounded in the present moment in time and location in space. Sense awareness does not spin off into the past and future like conceptual mind does. In fact, conceptual mind can only focus on the past or the future, for even if we are thinking about the present, by the time we have thought about it, it is gone. This is why our experience of conceptual consciousness feels so "heady" and unfulfilling.

However, when we open ourselves to our direct, nonconceptual experience of the here and now, we are nourished with fullness and insight. For example, earlier today, I was looking at some tiny flowers that are growing in the cracks of our patio. As I let go into the full experience of seeing these flowers, I felt more aware of their qualities: their pale lavender and white hue, their delicacy, and also their resilience as they grow out of the cracks in the cement. I felt a sense of their perkiness, and there were so many of them that I had a feeling of shared perkiness and upliftedness. This experience made me feel that I was anchored in and deeply connected with my world rather than just skating across its surface.

Such an experience does not have to involve something conventionally beautiful. We may feel the strength of a loud noise before we experience annoyance at being disturbed and try to figure out where the noise came from. In the first moment of nonconceptual experience, we may find that just the vivid experience of "loud" vibrates through our being, heightening and clarifying our awareness.

One powerful and wonderful way to work with nonconceptual experience is to open to whatever feelings are present now. We may conceptualize those feelings with labels such as boredom, inspiration, loneliness, nothingness, joy, tiredness, or excitement. But whatever label we apply, if we pay close attention, we see that the experience is much richer than anything a single word or phrase could possibly encompass.

Try just leaning into the experience without labels. When you have done that for a few minutes, you can try exploring the conceptual side for a bit by asking yourself what kind of loneliness this is. Maybe it is slightly tangy or bitter, maybe it has a quality of sharpness; it could be like a pinprick or a vast ocean, or a pinprick in a vast ocean. Then go back to the direct experience. Sometimes going back and forth between the conceptual and nonconceptual aspects helps us actually stay with a feeling and explore it further. When we become intimate with our own emotional lives, we learn more about ourselves and may even surprise ourselves with our capacity to feel, with the richness and subtlety of our emotional lives, and with our ability to transform stuck and painful places into fluid and meaningful ones.

In meditation, we train ourselves to come back to this nonconceptual experience and slow down the conceptual mind. This helps to calm the internal winds and bring them into balance in the body; this, in turn, eases feelings of anxiety and stress. As body and mind synchronize, awareness spreads evenly throughout the body.

Rebalancing conceptuality and nonconceptuality is greatly enhanced by silence. This is why meditation traditions encourage taking time to be in silence. Literal silence, as well as the move away from language, is important here. So we shut down our computers and avoid reading material and anything else related to words and language. As we stay in silence, we notice whole other areas of our being and ways of engaging in the world opening up.

They are always there, but conceptuality's volume is so high that we do not notice. Once the blare of conceptuality is turned down, the nonconceptual world emerges.

Reorienting ourselves to a state of balance between conceptual and nonconceptual experience can have surprising benefits. When we are actually open to our nonconceptual experience, it nourishes us fully. This helps to rectify all kinds of compulsive activity. For example, one reason we may eat compulsively is that we have disconnected from the quality of our experience and still feel the need to be fed, even though our bodies are not really hungry. When we fully connect with all five sensory experiences, we are truly nourished by our senses and no longer feel the need to keep eating beyond satiation. As our perceptions of the world open up and we see it more directly, it becomes vividly alive, wakeful, precise, and rich.

Making Time for Meditation Makes Time

A common obstacle that people find when beginning a meditation practice is the feeling that they do not have time to do it. This is one of the hallmarks of modern life; the cultural focus is on movement, speed, and accomplishment. We are then left feeling a lack of time and space. However, when we begin to engage with a meditation practice, we find that time expands. This is experientially true. Meditation actually gives us more time.

Through meditation, we slow down and become more mindful, and our ability to focus on a specific activity improves. Thus, we accomplish things more easily. This mindfulness makes us less prone to the little accidents that happen due to speediness and inattention. It also helps our relationships to be more harmonious. As we practice taking care of and developing friendliness toward ourselves, we find it easier to listen genuinely to others and to be kind and gentle. We all know how we behave when we feel stressed out, put-upon, and anxious and are holding ourselves to impossible ideals. As we grow kinder to ourselves and then to others, life flows more smoothly, and time feels less compressed.

This does not negate the reality of a busy life, but there are skillful methods for us to use in integrating meditation into our daily lives. While it is important to find time for formal meditation practice, when we can sit in a quiet place for a set period of time, we can also position "meditation cushions" throughout our day. When I was saving money to go to graduate school, I worked two full-time jobs, so meditation time was in short supply. One place I could usually be undistracted and quiet was the bathroom of the office where I worked. So I would meditate for a few minutes each time I went to the bathroom. Khenpo Rinpoche even calls the bathroom *gomkhang* (*sgoms khang*), which means "meditation room."

You can set up such places where you can touch base with your meditation practice throughout the day. Take a moment to pay attention to your breath or your felt sensations: when you first sit down in your car; before turning your computer on; as you fold the laundry; while you wait for the bus to arrive or the kettle to boil. Once you begin this integration of practice, you will probably spot many meditation opportunities.

When we begin a meditation practice, it is not that all difficulty suddenly evaporates from our lives, but we do find life more workable. That is why so many people who have started on the path of meditation have continued it throughout their lives.

7: How to Hold the Body

IN MEDITATION PRACTICE, we work with the interaction between body and mind. Holding the body in a particular posture encourages the mind to be alert yet focused. Holding the mind in a particular way encourages the body to be grounded yet wakeful. So we arrange both the body and the mind in ways that are conducive to the calm-abiding of both.

BODY POSTURE

Sometimes we mistakenly think of meditation as being, foremost, a mind practice. Actually, the body is so fundamental to meditation that the Tibetan master Dakpo Tashi Namgyal recommended meditating just by focusing on body posture:

> Body posture is important in all meditation practices, and is especially vital if one wants to bring mind to rest. Pay particular attention to it. Some find their minds are able to rest by following these instructions alone. If you first train in body posture for several days and nights, that would be excellent.[1]

The traditional meditation posture is called the Seven-Point Vairochana Posture. The nineteenth-century Tibetan master Dza Patrul Rinpoche, in *Words of My Perfect Teacher*, describes how, when the body is correctly aligned in this posture, the energy channels become aligned or straight. This allows the energy to run evenly and smoothly within the channels, helping mind to be "straight" as well. Our awareness feels easy and flowing rather than knotted or contracted.

THE SEVEN-POINT VAIROCHANA POSTURE

The following is a description of the classic Buddhist meditation posture, named for the buddha called Vairochana. The first point is the position of the legs. Traditionally, you sit on a cushion on the floor and cross your legs. However, if this position is difficult due to physical limitations or injury, then it is fine to sit on a chair with your feet flat on the floor. It is important that you use your lower body to create a solid foundation for your upper body. You should feel secure in your seated position. Whatever parts of your body are in contact with the floor, cushion, or chair feel as though they are rooting down, spreading into the earth. Encourage a sense of heaviness and relaxation in your lower body. This reflects your firm commitment to your meditation practice—you are not in a position from which you can easily leap up at the slightest impulse.

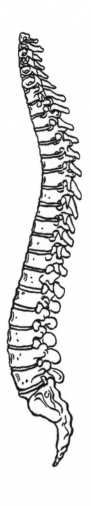

The second point is the placement of the hands. Allow your arms to hang naturally down at your sides; keep your elbows still; lift your hands and place them on your thighs. Keep your elbows in line with your shoulders so your arms do not reach forward or pull back. This prevents strain in the shoulders and arms. Your palms can be facedown on your knees. If you find that this encourages your shoulders to roll forward, you can try turning your palms upward with your fingers relaxed, creating a natural bowl shape.

The third point of the posture is the position of the spine. When you have a secure, grounded foundation, your spine is free to unfurl upward with your head floating on top. Stay

connected to the softness and fluidity of your body by maintaining
the natural curves of your spine.

Feel the openness of your heart area. You can try visualizing it as
a blooming lotus flower. This flower has no back or front: it keeps
opening and unfolding in all directions. This helps you to maintain
softness in the back of your body as well as the front.

If you are sitting in a chair, try not to lean back, but if you have
to, then support your back with cushions in a way that maintains
the natural curves of your spine. The most important point is to
keep your heart soft and open.

The fourth point is the position of the head and chin. Rather
than consciously tucking your chin, which, when overdone, can
create tension between your head and neck, feel that the crown of
your head is being drawn upward and allow this to create a small,
natural chin tuck. To get a sense of this, try pulling the hair at the
crown of your head, then pushing your chin forward, you will have
to exert effort to do this, because the natural movement is for your
chin to drop a little.

Daily activities often encourage us to jut our chin out, creating
a lot of tension in our shoulders, jaw, and neck. This tendency
is associated with being dissatisfied with ourselves in some way
and searching externally for satisfaction or a sense of self-worth.
By bringing awareness to this pattern (par-
ticularly when using a computer), we can
begin to reverse it, bringing both physical
and psychological benefits.

You can also try releasing your soft palate (the back of your throat just above the
tonsils) by making a guttural AH sound
and then gently closing your mouth. Feel
a bright, lifting sensation at the back of
your palate moving upward through the
crown of your head.

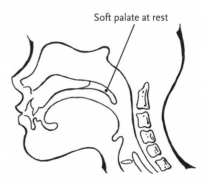

Soft palate at rest

The fifth point is the position of the shoulders. To place your shoulders in comfortable alignment, lift them slightly (which frees your chest) and take a few full, deep breaths. Feel your entire chest expand like a balloon. Then release your shoulders and scapulae down your back. Push down a little with your shoulders to counter the common tendency to lift them toward your ears—then release them. Allow your scapulae to flow gently down and slightly together. Your upper arms will naturally create an outward spiraling pattern, and your heart will lift.

The sixth point of the posture is the eye gaze. In general, your eyes remain open during meditation, with your gaze aimed a few feet in front of you. The focus is soft; you are not trying to look at anything in particular—your eyes are simply resting. If they feel strained, try extending your visual awareness to broaden your visual field, but do not move your gaze. When you practice with your eyes open, it helps you to be wakeful yet relaxed. You hold your attention where the internal and external worlds meet, without falling into one place or the other. You do not sink internally by shutting your eyes and disconnecting from your surroundings, which supports you in staying present, and you do not get distracted externally by looking around at objects, which supports you in focusing your mind. Practicing in this way also facilitates bringing meditation mind into daily life, as you will become used to meditating without shutting off from your environment.

If your eyes feel sore or dry, or your vision becomes fuzzy, you may be staring and have stopped blinking, so blink your eyes rapidly a few times. Then encourage them to be relaxed and natural.

If you find that your mind is distracted, you can try bringing your gaze closer in, lower your gaze, or even close your eyes completely to draw attention inward. If you feel sleepy or dull, try raising your gaze and taking in more of your environment. If you lift your gaze, make sure you do not tilt your head back, as this can cause tension in your neck and shoulders.

The seventh point is the placement of the tongue, which rests gently behind the upper teeth. Keep your lips relaxed, not pursed together; they can be slightly parted.

WORKING WITH THE NEEDS OF OUR INDIVIDUAL BODY

These guidelines for posture do not mean that you have to contort your body into an uncomfortable position in order to meditate. A skillful practitioner takes the basic guidelines and adapts them to his or her individual needs. If you need to sit on a chair, stand, or even lie down during your meditation session, that is fine. The most important thing is not to think that you cannot meditate because of your physical limitations.

A few years ago, I broke my foot just before going into retreat. I had to lie on my back with my foot elevated. Even in this position, it was still possible to align my body in a way that encouraged it to relax and remain wakeful. I propped one firm pillow behind my back so that my heart could stay open and another behind my head so that my spine aligned as it does in seated meditation but on a different plane. Then I raised my broken foot on a pillow in front of me.

This did not feel exactly the same as seated meditation, and at times I would get quite sleepy. But that was just something for me to work with in this situation. If you always wait for the ideal environment, physical health, or state of mind in order to meditate, you will probably wait a long time—possibly your entire life! In meditation, you are really learning to be with what is and work with what manifests in the moment. Meditation is extremely adaptable, and it is possible to meditate in any moment.

8: How to Hold the Mind

THE TRADITIONAL ANALOGY for working with the mind in meditation is that of training a horse. Initially, the mind is like a wild horse: it moves when it wants to, stops when it wants to, roams all over, and the best we can do is hold on and not get thrown off. When mind is wild, we cannot harness its raw power to any purpose. It can actually be quite destructive, creating a lot of chaos in our lives. Through meditation training, the wild horse of mind is tamed. The power is still there, but we have a way of harnessing it so that we can ride it with dignity and move in the direction we desire. In this way, we build a friendly relationship with mind, and it becomes our ally in life.

In meditation, mind focuses on an object, and there are many to choose from: physical sensations, the breath, or an object such as a candle or a stone. A simple object of focus is best, one that will not distract you too much and that feels calming. No judgment needs to be made about the object—it is simply there as a focus, an anchor for the mind. If you focus on your felt experience, go no further than simply being aware of it. If you focus on your breath, do not start analyzing it by thinking, "It feels constricted," "I'm not relaxed enough," "This isn't working," and so forth. Simply observe without judgment. When you get distracted by thoughts of the past or future, it is sufficient simply to recognize that you have been thinking—you can even silently label the thought "thinking" and then return to the object of focus.

As we practice, we play with the subtle border between

overexertion and lack of exertion, just like a musician tuning the strings of a guitar. If a string is too tight, it will snap; if it is too loose, it will not sound the note. As we apply the meditation technique, we do not try so hard that we are rigid and our mind is unable to rest naturally, and we are not so lax that we simply wander after every rippling thought or space out. We can consciously play with these two modes to fully familiarize ourselves with them and learn how and when to best employ discipline or relaxation. Then we become skillful meditators.

Initially, it may seem that you have a torrent of thoughts and the meditation seems to create more than usual. Most likely, it is not that your thoughts have suddenly increased but that you have started to notice them rather than just going along with them. Noticing the number of thoughts you have is actually a good sign; it means you are applying the meditation instructions. You may never have had the opportunity to see how much you think. As you progress with the meditation, you may use the labeling technique more subtly. Rather than actually labeling "thinking," you can simply return to the object. But if your mind is fuzzy and you are not sure when you are mindful or when you are distracted, then apply the labeling technique with more precision.

In meditation, we are working with reality. The reality of mind is that it is not one unchanging thing but rather a series of momentary consciousnesses arising and ceasing. Meditation happens in short flashes, not in our attempts to elongate the experience of calm-abiding. Practicing meditation regularly enables those flashes to occur more frequently, closer and closer together. This also means that, every moment, we have the possibility to drop into meditation. As the Tibetan master, the Lord of Yogis, Milarepa sings,

> Whenever you meditate on Mahamudra,
> Meditate in short sessions again and again.[1]

We are also encouraged to take breaks in our meditation practice. As Dakpo Tashi Namgyal puts it, "After your mind has settled down, then from within that relaxed, settled mind, and with a serene sense of joy, ease out of the practice and take a short rest. Keep your sessions short and frequent."[2]

If you sit down for a half hour of meditation and find during your session that your mind has become dull or agitated, then it is fine to take a short break from the technique. Allow your mind to rest without technique for thirty seconds or so, and then return to the practice with a refreshed mind.

Do not despair if you feel your meditation session has not gone well. If you are meditating regularly, then that is excellent. There is no need to judge your meditation. If you have an experience during practice that feels profound, do not try to recreate that experience in your next meditation session, as that is a sure way to avoid having it again! Just stay open to what is in the present moment of your experiential time and space.

TWO MAIN ENERGETIC PATTERNS IN MEDITATION

In terms of the subtle body, the two main energy patterns with which we work in meditation practice are the descending energy pattern and the ascending energy pattern. The descending pattern is the grounding sensation we feel particularly strongly through the lower body as our feet, thighs, and buttocks root firmly into the earth. We find a stable foundation for our body-mind in this pattern. As we pay closer attention, we also discover the descending pattern in our shoulders flowing down our back; in our hands resting on our knees; and in our jaw and earlobes melting downward, like stones gently sinking to the bottom of a lake.

Wherever we find the descending energy pattern, we find a

corresponding ascending pattern. The foundation of the seat and legs supports the ascending energy in the spine and center of the body. The energy lifts from the lower gate (see Closing the Lower Gate, page 104) through the center of the body. As the shoulders descend, they buoy up the heart, which floats on the central channel. As the earlobes and jaw flow downward, energy rises up through the soft palate and the crown of the head. Energy bubbles up through the center of the body like a fountain and cascades down on all sides.

One image I find particularly appealing for the energetic sensations experienced in seated meditation is the kelp seaweed that forms into extensive sea forests. It is firmly anchored to the ocean floor, like the rooting of our legs and seat that provides us with a firm ground so we do not get carried away with the tides. This rooting enables the seaweed to rise up through the water; as our spine unfurls upward, our head floats on top. The seaweed is surrounded by water, like the energetic field that surrounds our body and with which we are in constant communication. Sea forests provide rich habitats for all sorts of marine creatures, such as snails, fish, and mammals. Likewise, we have an immeasurable pantheon of felt sensations swimming around within us, from our toes to the tops of our heads.

In paying attention to our physical posture, we tune into all these more subtle experiences of energy. Rather than merely heaving this mound of flesh and bones into a particular position, we are accessing the felt experiences of our body and ever more subtle and profound qualities of our experience.

By working with these patterns, our body remains stable and erect but free of tension; it feels naturally at home. This encourages our mind to stay focused, awake, and simultaneously content and relaxed. While this is not so easily observable from the outside, our internal meditation experience is of a core connection to a continually flowing and unfolding stream of energy.

MOVEMENT AND STILLNESS IN
SEATED MEDITATION

Some techniques encourage us to remain perfectly still during meditation, with the mind focused one-pointedly on its object. This is useful in cutting off potential avenues of distraction. At the same time, the fluid internal energy may also distract us. So, particularly in the beginning, it can be helpful to focus on physical stillness.

It is important to know that you do not have to maintain your posture through excruciating pain; this would show little compassion for yourself. If you need to realign your posture and then return to stillness, that is fine, particularly if you have physical problems that need to be considered. As you develop your awareness and ability to focus, you may notice times when you are suspicious of your desire to move. You suspect it is not from a physical need but from a feeling of boredom or dullness. In noticing that, you have an opportunity to watch your mind. You may invite yourself to stay in the posture longer to see what happens.

The key point is that your attitude is never aggressive, and you always maintain a sense of self-care, exploration, and—most important—humor. Then you can more confidently explore the role of the energetic body in your meditation posture. Even in stillness, the body is in movement, and as you tune into the fluid energies in your body, more information about your posture is exposed to your awareness. You feel fine adjustments to your physical and subtle bodies unfold naturally. The process of meditation is a continual refinement, a back-and-forth between extremes: relaxation and alertness, tightness and looseness, overexertion and lack of exertion. In this way, you discover the center ground of physical, mental, and emotional balance.

Next, we will explore the meditation technique further using two different objects of focus—the breath and bodily sensations.

FOCUSING ON THE BREATH

The breath is an excellent focus for meditation because it is the meeting place of the full spectrum of human experience: the physical body, the subtle body, the mind, our emotional state, and our environment. As we breathe, we feel the physical body rise and fall. We feel the energetic body become invigorated and energized on the inhalations and relaxed and grounded on the exhalations. The mind tunes into the fluid nature of our existence, as the continually changing nature of the breath is immediately apparent (unlike focusing on a stone or statue, whose changeable nature is less obvious).

The breath is also a wonderful point of attention because it provides a direct reflection of our emotional state. For example, when we are tense or nervous, our breathing becomes shallow and concentrated in our upper body; we may even find we are barely breathing. When we are relaxed and happy, our breaths become deeper and longer. As we learn to observe the breath, we see how much information it holds about our current emotional state.

Lastly, our breathing is an oscillation between the external world and our internal environment. On the coarse level, oxygen from the outside world flows into the very core of our being, and carbon dioxide flows back out into the world. On a more subtle level, the movement and exchange is between internal and external energy, and we come to understand that there is really no difference between the two. There is only this one sea of energetic awareness.

David Gordon White (a widely studied scholar of and specialist in South Asian religions) describes this dynamic of the breath in the following way:

 [I]t is ultimately breath, breathing in and breathing out that unites the microcosm to the macrocosm. . . . The lunar months, solar years, etc. are so many temporal mesocosms, so many levels at which the human becomes joined to the absolute, through the bipolar dynamic of breathing in and breathing out.[3]

This breath is always available to us, but only in the present moment in time and location in space, so it holds us anchored in current reality. The breath is also a wonderful way to drop directly into the experience of how all things are constantly changing. Every place to which we may travel, object with which we interact, being to whom we relate, and even we ourselves have no permanence. This is true moment by moment.

Our common habit is to ignore this fluid quality of life and cling to things as being concrete and fixed. We freeze our world into solid blocks that are actually mere figments of our imagination. As we observe our breath closely, we experience each of its moments as completely unique. We enter the fluid nature of reality in a deeply profound yet palpable way. When we understand impermanence, we see the preciousness of every fleeting moment and every transient life. When we see the preciousness of life, we realize that everything is worthy of our attention. And we learn to give this close attention to our precious lives through meditation.

HOW TO WORK WITH THE BREATH

There are various instructions for how to focus on the breath. Initially, it can be helpful to count each round (the inhalation and exhalation are one round). You can count to ten or twenty-one and then start again at one. This can be particularly helpful when your mind is distracted and a lot of thoughts are coming up. It provides a strong anchor for mind's attention.

If you find you easily maintain this focus, you can simply concentrate on the breath coming in and going out. When you find that you have wandered off into thought, label that "thinking," without placing any judgment on what you were thinking. You even apply the technique of nonjudgment when you are unable to be nonjudgmental.

Do not be seduced away from practice to either scribble down some insight you have or to berate yourself for the unwholesome and degraded areas that your mind has fallen into. While writing this book, I spent part of my time in retreat, alternating between seated meditation, movement meditation, and writing. Sometimes, during meditation, I would come up with ideas for the book and be tempted to reach for my computer. Then I would ask myself, "Do you want to live a life committed to a path of transformation, or do you just want to write about?" So now those pearls of wisdom are lost to the world! Fortunately, genuine wisdom usually finds a way to bubble up somewhere, somehow.

All your thinking in meditation practice is just thinking. Label it as such and return to the breath. If you feel more settled in the state of calm-abiding and the "thinking" label feels too heavy, when you notice subtle flickers of thought, you can simply come back to the breath without using the label. The instruction from Dakpo Tashi Namgyal is, "Exert just enough effort so that mind does not elaborate ideas or move to some outer distraction. Let mind naturally abide."[4]

Meditation on Bodily Sensations

Another way to focus the mind is to hold your attention on the experiences of the body. Place your body on the meditation seat and let it rest, then place your mind on your body and let it rest. Simply notice what is occurring in the felt experience of your body by opening awareness to it. Do not apply judgments or add narrative for what you are feeling. Do not think of ways to fix it or maintain it; just notice the sensation and let it be. Actually paying attention to your body without it having to cry out with disease or injury to get your attention may be a new experience. It is surprising how little real attention we give our bodies, our living homes.⟩

Like the breath, the body is a constantly changing, fluid entity. We can experience this by focusing on bodily sensations in meditation.

Sit in your meditation posture and just become aware of what is happening in your body. Feel the sensation directly without adding any label, like "lightness" or "heaviness," "pain" or "pleasure." You do not need to examine your experience further, wondering if the pain in your side is due to that sandwich you had for lunch or whether you should do something about that sensation in your throat. Those are valid thoughts, but they are for another time. Do not allow thoughts to proliferate based on your sensations. Touch the experience, let it go, and see what arises in the next moment.

Even when we think a sensation lasts for a few moments, we find on subtler analysis that each moment is similar to the others but not exactly the same. We never find the exact point where pleasure turned to pain or when a sensation arose or ceased. Just as when we watch the breath, each moment is unique, although we may call them all "breathing."

When you feel your mind has wandered, which it does, know you have wandered, invigorate your awareness, and return to sensations. You may want to bring a little energy into sensing your body at this point so that it regains your attention. Sometimes taking a few deep breaths into your lower belly can help. Then just settle back into awareness of sensations.

How to Structure a Meditation Session

It is good to have an environment that is conducive for meditation—one that is tidy and uplifted. If this is impossible for whatever reason, it is best to practice regardless of environment. You do not necessarily need a dedicated space, but you can sanctify the space each time you practice by tidying it or placing a candle or flower somewhere. You can think of this as an offering to the sacredness at the heart of your daily life experience. A mind of self-respect and clarity naturally cares for its environment. And when you respect and beautify your outer world, you feel more wholesome and healthy internally.

If you want to meditate for a particular length of time, using a timer may spare you from having to check the clock constantly. Five minutes of meditation spent looking at a clock is a lot longer than five minutes of meditation spent meditating. After some practice, you may be more internally aware of the time and not need to rely on a timer or clock.

A good way of preparing the body and mind for meditation is to do three cleansing breaths. (You will find full instructions for this on page 110.) Before sitting down, move your body around a little to loosen it up. This will help you ease into a comfortable sitting posture. Then begin with some lower belly breaths (explained on page 113) to help ground you in the present moment and location and to ground awareness in the center of your body. As you perform the belly breaths, you can also rest your awareness in your bodily sensations. Be aware of how your posture feels. Feel into the subtleties of your body's alignment. Feel its energetic quality. You can either continue to focus on bodily sensations for part or all of your session or begin to focus on your breath.

Once your session has finished, you can close it with a sense of gratitude for your ability to have such a session. Then dedicate the positive energy of your practice in some way; offer it out to benefit the greater world. You may want to use the dedication verse on page 154.

If you ever feel lost in your meditation and are not sure how to coordinate the whole thing, forget the instructions and return to simplicity. Remember to "just be." Feel how those words resonate in your being. When you apply too much instruction, you contract and get tense; you cannot find any internal openness; space shuts

down. When that happens, simply rest and be. It can also be helpful
to read Milarepa's lines on meditation experience:

> Do you know how to rest your mind?
> If you don't know how to rest your mind
> Without thoughts jumping all around
> Let your mind rest uncontrived
> Rest with a child's independence
> Rest like an ocean free of waves
> Rest with a candle flame's clarity
> Rest like a corpse, without arrogance
> Rest like a mountain, so still
> There simply is no name for what mind is really like.[5]

PART THREE
Extending Practice

9: Using Adversity to Enhance the Practice of Buddhist Yoga

ONCE YOU HAVE an established meditation practice, you can begin to extend that practice into other areas of your life, even the parts you find challenging. The view of Buddhist yoga is that adversity can be your friend on the path of practice, for suffering gives you a strong incentive to find some deeper meaning to your life, some deeper place of being. You long to free yourself from your suffering and rediscover your true nature and innate good qualities. This is why Milarepa sang, "Adversity has been very kind to me."[1]

This does not mean that he reached a point where he could no longer distinguish his feelings and was unable to understand what suffering felt like. But through his training, he gave up struggling with what was occurring. Whatever arose for him, he could rest within that experience without rejecting it or trying to get rid of it. Recognizing that experiences naturally change and dissolve, he was free from grasping at or trying to hold on to anything.

Difficult situations are often times of intense sensation. This provides a ground for strongly connecting with our present experience, which is essential on the path to joining with our true nature. As Trungpa Rinpoche explained,

> It is just that pain is pain and it makes you awake. . . .
> When you are really sick, it is the most healthy situation you have experienced, because you really do have a

connection with your body and your mind at the same time. You really feel there, completely there.[2]

Not only are our adverse experiences beneficial for our own path, but they are the best way for us to connect with others. Suffering is a universal experience. This is why the Buddha chose suffering as the first topic of his teachings. So when we connect with our own suffering, we can also recall that many beings all over the world are having similar experiences. This helps us develop understanding, love, and compassion for others.

WORKING WITH SICKNESS

The renowned Tibetan yogi Gyalwa Gotsangpa[3] endured severe and lengthy illnesses, among them an imbalance of wind energy, which produces symptoms similar to what we would now call an anxiety disorder. Gotsangpa persevered by meditating on the true nature of his illness, and he achieved profound realization as a result. He sang many songs about how to take illness to the yogic path. Here is one verse from such a song:

> The illness and its painfulness have neither base nor root
> Relax into it, fresh and uncontrived
> Revealing Dharmakaya way beyond all speech and
> thought
> Don't shun them, pain and illness are basically good.[4]

We can learn how to practice Gotsangpa's method by studying the meaning of this verse. The first line describes how illness and the suffering it causes do not truly exist. How can we know that sickness is not real? Because, as Gotsangpa says, it has no basis where it exists, no root or origin from which it comes. If we look at the body, we do not find "sickness"; we find cells that are made of atoms, atoms that are made of smaller particles that are in turn made of even smaller particles—ultimately, we cannot even find the tiniest particle of matter in the body. There is no root or basis for sickness in a body that is not actually made of any particles of matter.

If we look at the mind, we do not find sickness there either. We may find a thought ("I'm sick," or "I'm in pain"), but if we ask ourselves what that experience of sickness and pain is actually like, we quickly run out of words to describe it. For example, we may start by describing a dull ache. What is that like? It may be slightly heavy and dense or knotted. But the further we go with our questioning, we find that conceptual terms cannot really describe our experience. All we find is inexpressible and luminous awareness that is the true nature of all thoughts and emotions. We find no entity that can ultimately be described as "sickness."

Much of the suffering we experience when we are ill does not come from the direct experience itself but from our conceptualizing about our experience and our struggle with the reality of our situation. One mistaken concept we have is believing that we and our sickness truly exist. We can understand this by imagining how different we would feel if we knew we were in a dream and neither the sickness nor we were real. The experience would not necessarily disappear, but we might find more relaxation and a lighter touch to our experience of illness. We would probably still prefer the illusory appearances of health, but we would not need to compound our suffering by believing our sickness to be a permanent and fixed reality.

This probably sounds like a challenging way to approach sickness, and it is! However, if we practice with sickness in stages, then we will find it easier to reach the profound level of practice that realizes the lack of inherent existence in our condition or any other experience. When we are sick, we often constrict our thinking around this experience and add many layers of struggle and dissatisfaction. Not only do we feel unwell, but we also think,

"This is always happening to me. I was sick like this last year, and here it is again. Just last week I had that cold, and now this! It's just one thing after another. I probably won't make it to that important meeting next week. This is never-ending."

All of this thinking increases our suffering and discomfort. To begin with, let us see if we can just let these voices trail off a little. Our calm-abiding meditation practice aids us in this process. When we have practiced being with the fleeting nature of thoughts that arise in our meditation, we grow more familiar with our mind's activities so that it becomes easier for us to simply be with difficult thoughts when they arise and rest in the stillness beneath those thoughts.

Having calmed these upsetting thought patterns, we can begin to be really present with the current experience of sickness. This is the next step—just being with the physical sensations that arise, with a sense of curiosity about our felt experience. We take the approach of "This is what is happening for me now, so let me be present to it, be awake for it." Instead of trying to alter or block our experience, we apply deep, open listening to connect with what is there. In this way, we develop a friendly relationship with our mind and its experience; we do not reject certain parts of mind's experience. Just this simple technique can transform how we experience illness.

When we have developed a friendlier and more open relationship with our experience, we can begin to go deeper, to examine what is really going on. If we look for some truly existent sickness or person who experiences sickness, we find no such things. Nothing in the entire world or in all our experience is solid, fixed, perma-nent, or unchanging. All we find in reality is a pure experience of basic awareness.

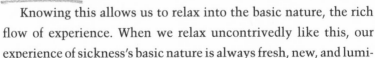

Knowing this allows us to relax into the basic nature, the rich flow of experience. When we relax uncontrivedly like this, our experience of sickness's basic nature is always fresh, new, and lumi-

The absolute basis of reality, from which all phenomena emanate.

nous. In fact, it is nothing but the enlightened essence of mind, Dharmakaya beyond thought and expression. Therefore, there is no reason to shun pain or illness, because their nature is pure.

When you are sick, it is helpful to sing Gotsangpa's verse, meditate on its meaning, and think, "This is like being sick in a dream when I know I am dreaming." Think of your body, particularly the part that is sick, as being appearance-emptiness—free of particles of matter, perfectly pure, like a dream body or a rainbow. Let your mind relax in its own basic nature of inexpressible awareness. By using these methods, sickness leads to joining with naturalness, and you discover how sickness is your friend on the path.

It is worth emphasizing that these teachings on sickness's lack of true existence are an invitation to explore our own experience (should we choose to take it) and not a method for engaging someone else's sickness. The last thing a sick person needs to hear from us is, "Your sickness is not real." This teaching is the most profound and subtle view and cannot be captured in such a simplistic statement. It also does not propose that all sickness is psychosomatic. Everything we experience is not real. We can use meditation to cultivate our mind, but that does not mean an uncultivated mind is at fault when we get sick! Again, reality is far too complex and subtle for simplistic statements like that.

Yogic Movement Methods to Aid Healing

There are also specific methods for working with sickness and healing in yogic movement. While allowing your mind to relax in a meditative state, do some easy exercise with the sick part of your body if you are able. Moving that part of your body, even in a subtle way, is beneficial. If you cannot move physically, you can focus your mind on the sick part of your body and feel its natural, internal movement. Bring full awareness to the parts of the body you are working with and visualize your body going through the exercises. This same method can be used when you are traveling and in confined spaces for long periods of time. If it is possible to move your body subtly, you can do that, but if not, just visualize the exercises while paying close attention to the feeling in your body.

Another method is to think of the sick or injured part of your body as being pure and open space. For example, if you have stomach problems, visualize your stomach area as vast, empty space. This is a powerful method for reversing the contraction you usually experience around a painful body part and the tendency to concentrate too much on that area.

You can also work on focusing the internal winds in the afflicted part of your body. The winds of the energetic channels in the subtle body (explained in chapter 5) contain healing energy. These winds naturally gather wherever you focus your mind, and it is possible to use this energy in the healing process. Hold your attention on the ailing part of your body and breathe into it. The healing wind energy will naturally flow there. Just be gentle with the practice, and do not overexert yourself.

When you combine this method with movement, it has even greater potency. The Dance of the Warriors exercise (see page 117) is good for this practice because, once you are familiar with it, it has a flowing, rhythmic ease. While performing the exercise, focus your attention on the sick or injured part of your body. If you feel generally under the weather, you can simply apply this technique to the energy centers along the central channel: the crown, throat, heart, origin point, and lower gate. Start at the top and gradually move down through the energy centers. Once you have reached the lower gate, you can go up the chain again, spending a few minutes in each location. As you do this, maintain some awareness of your whole body but concentrate most of it on the current focal point.

It is important to remember that these skillful means for working with sickness are complementary to, rather than substitutes for, remedies prescribed by doctors or other medical practitioners.

WORKING WITH FEAR

Various practices in Tibetan Buddhism are specifically designed to help us work with fear. This is one way to find out exactly how far our practice has progressed. When we are enjoying a cup of tea and life is good, mind seems calm and we feel that we are doing well. But in challenging or threatening situations, mind may not be so stable.

In Tibet, practitioners went to charnel grounds where dead bodies were left to be consumed by vultures. They would practice in these terrifying places as a way to work with their most fearful states of mind. Khenpo Rinpoche lived and practiced in charnel grounds; to confront fear and repulsion, he would even wear the clothes of the dead.

After coming to the West, he found other skillful methods for confronting fear—he would go to amusement parks. The rides that shake you around and tip you up and down offer a wonderful opportunity for vivid experiences of fear. When the emotion arises, you meditate by simply looking directly at the sensation of fear. Khenpo Rinpoche particularly enjoyed Universal Studios and the virtual-reality ride called Back to the Future, where you are apparently flying in space and then seem to be diving down, but in reality, you are not going anywhere. You may have vivid experiences, but none of it is really happening. The more you can remember the dreamlike, illusory quality of appearances, the easier it is to relax with what is. The practice is then to apply this view to your dreamlike, illusory daily life.

One of the events many of us fear most is our own death. Through working with adversity and particularly with fear, we gain confidence that bolsters our ability to face whatever life has in store for us, even if that is the apparent end of this individual life.

The Indestructible Vajra Posture (page 148) exercise specifically helps us with the death experience. At the time of death, we will likely be afraid and experience uncomfortable physical sensations. This posture can be physically demanding and hard to hold for a long period—when we do, it gives rise to intense sensations. Khenpo Rinpoche would sometimes keep us in this posture for long periods, which led to the strong desire to do something else—anything else. When death comes, we will probably have other plans for that time; it is unlikely to be marked on the calendar as an event for the day. By holding the Indestructible Vajra Posture, we develop the ability to relax and surrender to what is in this moment, even when it is an uncomfortable sensation. Training in this way will likely be a great asset to us at the time of death.

One important point to remember is that even while we have strong sensations, there is no truly existent self to die, no truly existent body for us to be separated from. When the Sixteenth Karmapa,[5] Rangjung Rigpe Dorje, was in the hospital dying of cancer, he said, "Nothing happens." Even at the moment many of us most fear, he could see the illusory, dreamlike nature of death. To relax with reality even at this time, we need to train in these methods while we have the opportunity.

WORKING WITH LAZINESS AND TIREDNESS

Existence and peace are equality
Free from all conceptuality
So striving and straining to accomplish some goal—
Oh, what a tiring thing to do![6]
—DOMBE HERUKA

The first thing we need to do with laziness is to correctly identify whether what we are addressing is laziness or actually physical or mental exhaustion. This is a crucial point and not to be glossed over quickly. Nowadays, we are often encouraged to work with tiredness and sickness in very unskillful ways. It is considered commendable to push the body to its limits, to power through any discomfort, sickness, or unpleasant physical sensations we may have. We are told laudatory stories of business tycoons or political leaders who keep up a tremendous work rate and rarely get more than three hours of sleep a night. We are offered all types of cold cures, herbs, and energy drinks and bars that will get us back to work and keep us there relentlessly, regardless of what our felt experience is or what our body-mind needs.

We can take medications and herbal remedies to wake us up and others to send us to sleep. We do this rather than find intelligent approaches to balancing the mind and finding a more stable and satisfying solution to working with rest and activity. Somehow we have become so disconnected from bodily experience that we override any warning signs of the need to slow down and listen to what our body is expressing.

Khenpo Rinpoche often spoke of the need to work with our laziness, to exert ourselves vigorously in these exercises. It is definitely important for us to apply ourselves with exertion and continuity in our activities in order to reap the benefits. However, we need to really look at this point with subtlety so that we are not using the technique to increase our speediness and disconnection with our bodily experience. In the modern world, many people are struggling with chronic fatigue and various forms of burnout, overwork, and tiredness. We need to be alert to these dangers.

Grounding our movement practice in the preliminary exercises where we feel into our embodied experience helps us open this internal communication. When we really listen to our own body, we will know how far we can take the exercise in this moment: whether we need a vigorous or more relaxed session, whether we should do a long or short session, whether we should test our limits or back off a bit, whether we should focus more on the meditation or the movement. We each know ourselves better than anyone else possibly can, and the more we open up this communication with our body, the more insight we will gain. Then every session will be uniquely tailored to our individual needs in the moment, which will keep our practice fresh, alive, and powerfully connected to the qualities of wisdom and compassion.

On the occasions when we feel we have correctly identified that we are being lazy rather than simply exhausted, one method we can apply is to look for the laziness we are experiencing. We can ask ourselves, "Is it really my body being lazy, or is it my mind?" We think we feel laziness in the body, but when we look at the body, we know that conventionally it is just made of atoms. Atoms do not experience any sense of laziness.

The Buddhist teachings tell us the body is not even made of atoms. When we analyze, we do not find any small particle of physical material that comprises the body. Gradually, through examining our self and our world, we understand that the body is just pure wisdom-awareness, like a body of light or a rainbow. It appears to exist, but it is not truly existent. This leads us to understand even more fully how no sense of laziness can come from the body.

Understanding this, you can play with the limits of your energy. If you feel lazy or tired when practicing, try meditating on your body being a body of light; see if that lightness then enters your experience of your body and diminishes your tiredness. Sense your dreamlike body fluidly moving in a dreamlike world.

But do not push your body in a way that will cause physical harm and increase mental aggression. While bodies are dreamlike, they can still experience dreamlike injury and harm. But you can play with really listening to your body and seeing where your laziness is coming from. Ask yourself, "How can I work with this? Is the best method to really listen and be compassionate with the current condition of my body? Or is the laziness coming from mental boredom or malaise?"

The Third Karmapa, Rangjung Dorje, wrote about recognizing

everything to be of the nature of wisdom. When we rest the mind naturally in this view and see thoughts and appearances that arise as wisdom, then we are not so prone to laziness. Whatever activity we are engaged in, if we know the nature of thoughts and feelings as they arise, they do not have the same effect on us.

Another method you can apply when feeling lazy is to work with the lower gate. If you are not accustomed to doing this, try the Toning the Lower Gate exercise (see page 115). When you feel tired, gently close the lower gate. This holds the subtle energies within the body and powers up the central channel and the ascending energy. Because this is a subtle method, you can apply it whenever you wish, and no one will know what you are up to—unless they see your hair stand on end.

When I was traveling with Khenpo Rinpoche in Italy, he had me memorize all the root verses of various sutras. I had to do this in the evening as we were in a teaching retreat, so I was getting very little sleep. I would sometimes fall asleep in the teachings. So Rinpoche instructed me to close the lower gate at these times and gave me a secret signal in the teachings when he saw me beginning to doze off. It worked quite well . . . most of the time!

WORKING WITH PROCRASTINATION

Khenpo Rinpoche gives two excellent pieces of advice to help us when we have difficulty even getting to our practice:

Let body take control of the mind.
Let mind take control of the body.[7]

Sometimes our mind overthinks and paralyzes us; we cannot see a way forward into action, and we avoid what we are trying to do by allowing our mind to be distracted by other things. At such times, we can try dropping all mental activity and surrendering to the body. For this moment, we let the mind and concepts go. We let our body take whatever action it needs to get to the practice space and begin moving. Then we allow our body to feel its way into the movement, just as we discussed earlier. We do not force the movement from the outside; we feel into it. Even though our mind may think our body does not want to exercise, there is always natural energy in the body. We can try asking our body, "If you were to move, in which way would you move?"

Let your style of movement be dictated by your body. Begin with the first exercise and allow your body to enter into it in whatever manner feels right—energetically, fluidly, softly, or strongly. There are always patterns of movement in your body, so just surrender to the natural pattern of its energy without trying to force it to do anything.

When you move your body, your mind naturally has a focus, and it has less desire to follow thoughts that create difficulties and unpleasant feelings for you. Once you have simply begun by trusting your body's natural movement, it is much easier to continue. You ease your way into the practice by following your body there.

The second instruction, "Let mind take control of the body," seems to negate the first instruction, but sometimes we need one thing and other times we need the opposite. When we think of the reasons for doing something, we are much more likely to undertake it. It is helpful to increase our motivation by recalling the benefits of practice, remembering sessions we have enjoyed and felt good about afterward, and thinking about the pleasure of moving our body. If we need more inspiration, we can also read over sections of this book or find other methods that encourage and inspire us in our practice.

These two instructions help to get us to the practice and keep both the body and mind flexible.

WORKING WITH ANXIETY

When we feel anxious or agitated, exercising with vigor is highly beneficial for our subtle body. This is because anxiety often locks itself in the subtle body in a frozen energy pattern. This can occur anywhere in the body but often manifests in the stomach, the heart center, or the throat center. It can be difficult to sit with such a feeling, and moving the body may be more efficacious in easing the stress. Performing these exercises or even going for a brisk walk can help to release the energy.

Khenpo Rinpoche describes how practitioners who had spent a long time in retreats in mountain caves would sometimes get uptight and find it difficult to relax. When this happened, the yogis or yoginis would go on pilgrimage. They would walk long distances, moving their bodies vigorously every day. Sometimes practitioners would walk for many months, and as a result, their minds and bodies would become more relaxed and spacious.

When you are anxious, your body contracts and becomes rigid, the channels get knotted, and the wind energies get stuck. Moving your body loosens up all of these uncomfortable patterns. Your physical body is soothed, and the wind energies flow more easily. Your mind then feels more relaxed, buoyant, and spacious.

Traditionally, in Tibet, the Four-Limb Exercise (page 133) was considered particularly helpful when practitioners suffered from anxiety, stress, or mental tension. This exercise and its corresponding visualization help release stuck energy and shift pent-up negativity, and was considered especially good for people who studied a lot. Being hunched over books for long periods can compress the internal winds in the upper body and give rise to anxiety and tension. Meditators who sat still for long periods of time and developed similar feelings of anxiety and tension also practiced this exercise. In the modern world, those of us who spend long hours in front of a computer are also prone to this kind of discomfort and can greatly benefit from this exercise.

The Wet Wooly Sheep Shake Out (page 125) is also wonderful for releasing anxiety. Just as a good cry can release tension and anxiety, simply shaking or vibrating the body releases frozen energy. We see this natural remedy used particularly by small animals, like rabbits. They maintain a high level of vigilance, constantly looking out for eagles, dogs, or other kinds of predators. This creates tension in the body, and it is not unusual to see rabbits suddenly leap into the air or shake out their whole bodies.

When you feel anxious, you can try either of these exercises, or if you feel like a more free-form remedy, go for a brisk walk or simply leap and shake like a wild rabbit.

10: Practicing with Syllables and Song

In Buddhist yogic exercise, there is a verbal component to the practice as well as a physical one, most often in the form of songs or syllables. The tradition of singing began with Shakyamuni Buddha. One of the twelve categories of teachings given by the Buddha is the "Set of Teachings Given in Melody," which he sang to his students.

Khenpo Rinpoche often begins yogic practice sessions with a song by the Lord of Yogis, Milarepa, who is renowned for the thousands of profound songs of realization he composed spontaneously. Milarepa would sing these songs to his students, strangers, his family, animals wandering in the mountains—anyone who would listen.

One of the benefits of singing is that profound songs are much easier to memorize than long teaching texts; through song, we internalize the Dharma teachings. Singing also has a highly beneficial effect on the body-mind. On the physical level, it makes us breathe deeply and expand our lungs. On the subtle level, singing in a clear voice opens the subtle channels and allows the energies to flow smoothly. And on the mind level, it can really cheer us up.

The song Khenpo Rinpoche chose as a warm-up to the yogic exercise sessions is Milarepa's *Eighteen Kinds of Yogic Joy*[1]:

> I bow at the feet of the genuine guru
> Because of merit gathered, I've met this lord

The guru with his prophecy is what has brought me here
My comfortable castle, this wooded mountain range
This is a meadowland so beautiful in bloom
The trees are dancing in the midst of all the trees

This is a place of play, where the monkeys and the
    langurs play
A place where birds speak in birdlike tongues
A land of flying bees on gentle wings
Where day runs into night, and rainbow paintings shine
Summer runs into winter, a light drizzle falls
Autumn runs into springtime, the mist comes rolling in

In a solitary place like this, I the yogi Milarepa
Am feeling very clear, light, well, meditating on
    emptiness mind
When I get a lot of stuff coming up, I feel extremely well
When the highs roll into lows feels even better still
Feels so good to be a human being without the karmic deeds
When confusion gets complicated, I feel extremely well

Fearsome visions getting worse and worse feels even
    better still
Kleshas, birth and death and freedom from those is a good
    way to feel
With the bullies getting worse and worse, I feel extremely
    well
When there's not a painful illness in sight feels even
    better still
The suffering being bliss, feels so good that feeling bad
    feels good
Since the trulkhor comes from what I am, it feels
    extremely good

To leap and run about is dance, feels even better still
To be a king of speech with a treasury of song feels good
That the words are like the buzzing of bees feels
    extremely good
That the sound it makes is merit-collecting feels even
    better still
The bliss is good in the expanse of the confidence of
    strength of mind
What develops on its own by its own force feels
    extremely good

What comes out looking like a hodgepodge feels even
    better still
This happy experience song by a yogi carefree
Is for you who believe in what you're doing here
To take along with you when you go[2]

This song was originally sung to five female practitioners who visited Milarepa while he was in retreat at Tiger Cave Lion Fortress in Yolmo, Nepal. It starts with Milarepa expressing his devotion to his teacher, Marpa the Translator. Then he describes the environment, the animals, and the weather with great appreciation. Milarepa observes everything in the phenomenal world—it is all worthy of his close attention. He goes on to describe his own experiences and how they are blissful, even though some of them sound like situations that we would usually think of as uncomfortable or miserable.

What enables Milarepa to perceive "bullies" and "confusion" as blissful is his practice of meditation on "emptiness mind." Having seen that his difficulties are not solidly existent, his experience of them is workable. When we give up struggling against our experience, we relax. Within that relaxation is true bliss—the bliss of abandoning the struggle.

The way to move when singing this song is described in the line, "Since the trulkhor comes from what I am, it feels extremely good." *Trulkhor* (*'phrul 'khor*) is the term for physical yogic exercise that is taught in the Vajrayana ("adamantine vehicle," the set of Mahayana practices that is kept secret), and it involves many specific movements. However, what Milarepa describes here is natural trulkhor. Another way of translating this line is, "The natural expression of my experience is yogic exercises, so I am happy." This describes the process whereby through naturally resting the mind within itself, the meditational experiences of bliss, clarity, and nonconceptuality arise. Then by resting within that experience and moving your body, you spontaneously perform natural yogic exercise, and that feels good.

So you sing the song, leave your mind settled within itself, and move your body in natural ways that feel good.

THE SYLLABLE AH

The syllable AH is often used in these exercises, and when practicing in a group, it is the signal to change the movement and go in the opposite direction. AH has significance for various reasons. In Tibetan and Sanskrit, it is considered the root of all language, because all consonants in those languages inherently have the sound AH. Symbolically, this syllable has a universal quality. It is a part of everything, just as the reality of emptiness is a part of everything. So AH is also considered to be the sound of emptiness. This is the sound we make when we are born, when we make love, and when we die.

When saying this syllable, the sound comes from the back of the throat. This releases the soft palate, which connects you to the subtle body and the top of the central channel. As you utter this syllable, allow your earlobes to descend; release your jaw; and feel the bright, lifting sensation in your soft palate. As you finish, bring your lips together softly, rest your tongue behind your teeth, and feel a gentle inner smile, as if you were a connoisseur of syllable sounds.

As you make this sound, look at its essence, which is impermanence and emptiness; there is nothing permanent and graspable in sound. Having looked directly at this essence, rest within experiential awareness; simply feel.

Khenpo Rinpoche wrote these verses on how to practice with the syllable AH:

> Ah is unborn,
> So rest in the realm of unborn emptiness.
>
> Ah is unceasing
> So rest in the realm of unceasing luminosity.
>
> Ah is free of fabrication,
> So rest in the realm free from fabrications.
>
> Ah is great bliss
> So rest in the realm of inseparable bliss-emptiness.[3]

THE SOUND OF LAUGHTER

The syllables HA HA and HEE HEE are also important in these exercises, particularly in the exercise Dance of the Warrior Laughing at Appearances (page 137). These are the sounds of laughter. Using these syllables helps bring us into the lower belly, just like a deep belly laugh. In the West, we have the aphorism "Laughter is the best medicine," and modern scientific research[4] is beginning to catalog the health benefits of laughter. Also, as our temperature rises during physical exercise, making these sounds helps expel excess heat from the body.

Khenpo Rinpoche's nuns in Bhutan choreographed a dance to his autobiographical song "The Sky Dragon's Profound Roar," which concludes with these lines:

HA HA! Dechen Rangdrol's[5] conduct that's attachment-free
A HO! It's time to fly in the expanse of sky of spacious
    Mother[6]

At this point in the dance, the nuns lean back with their hands on their bellies in a great belly laugh. In Bhutan, when we would sing this for Khenpo Rinpoche, he would join in the dance at this point, as he really enjoyed the laughter gesture. Rinpoche often includes the syllables HA HA, HEE HEE, and HO HO in his compositions.

TIBETAN VICTORY CRY

In the Warrior Lunge (page 139), we use the syllables KI KI SO SO. These syllables begin the traditional Tibetan cry, *"Ki ki so so lha gyello!"* which means, "Victory to the deities!" This cry is often shouted in exuberant delight upon reaching a mountain's summit. It is an exclamation of victory and strength, and that is how we use it in this exercise—with great internal confidence and vigor. In Tibetan, this is called *lungta* (*rlung rta*), or "windhorse," referring to our innate qualities of energy, fearlessness, and fortitude.

11: Practice in Daily Life

Going, wandering, sleeping, resting—I look at mind
This is virtuous practice without sessions or breaks.[1]
—MILAREPA, THE LORD OF YOGIS

YOGIC PRACTICE encompasses not only exercise, singing, and laughing, but all of life's activities; the more we bring the yogic attitude to all we do, the more benefit we will reap. Modern life can be so fast-paced, busy, and demanding that it is easy for us to feel like we do not have enough time to meditate. However, Buddhist yoga is ideally incorporated into our daily activities. By briefly reflecting on renunciation, bodhichitta, and the profound view from time to time during the day, we blend practice and daily life. We train in acting without attachment but with compassion and bodhichitta, as well as with certainty in the view—complete willingness to be with the naked reality of whatever is happening in a given situation. This allows practice to flow continually rather than confining it to meditation sessions.

The only obstacle to joining with the naturalness of the appearances of daily life is the habit of solidifying the world, of thinking things are fixed in the way we perceive them in this moment. The heavier our solidification, the more we separate ourselves from the natural flow of reality and the more narrow-minded and agitated we become. To help us counteract that tendency, the Buddha taught the practice of the "illusion-like samadhi"[2] (the state of undistracted concentration that sees everything, including distracting

thoughts and sensory objects, to be like an illusion) in verses like
this one from *The Sutra of the Noble Collection*:

> All the images conjured up by a magician—
> The horses, elephants, and chariots in his illusion,
> Whatever may appear there, know that none of it is real,
> And it's just like that with everything there is.[3]

Khenpo Rinpoche revised the first two lines to make them more
applicable for modern practitioners:

> All the images conjured up by a director—
> The cities, cars, and airplanes, everything that's in the movies,
> Whatever may appear there, know that none of it is real,
> And it's just like that with everything there is.

Khenpo Rinpoche regularly sings verses like this one as he goes
about his daily life, and he frequently composes his own sponta-
neous verses as well, such as this one that he sang while swimming
in the ocean:

> In this illusory ocean,
> A dreamlike person,
> Swims like a water-moon,
> And crosses over into equality's expanse.[4]

We can adapt this verse for all the different activities we undertake. For example,

> In this illusory grocery store,
> A dreamlike person,
> Stands in line like in a movie,
> And crosses over into equality's expanse.

Equality's expanse is the true nature of reality, in which dualistic differences, distinctions, and contradictions do not exist. All such differences are equally dreamlike and illusory (appearance-emptiness), and we cross over into equality's expanse when we see this. Even the activities that we consider spiritual or mundane are equality. In fact, there is no such distinction. Every moment of our experience is valuable, worthy of close attention, and an opportunity to remember equality and join again with naturalness.

To understand and implement this, we must ensure that we avoid the temptation to create an alternative version of reality, an imagined "Buddhist" reality. This happens if we disavow, cover over, or nullify our own direct experience with ideas like, "I am not a truly existent being, so there is no need to pay attention to my experience," or "I can just say this experience is empty and do not need to examine or work with it any further." The Buddha warned that the potential danger here is to use the teachings on emptiness to avoid having to deal with the uncomfortable aspects of life. That disconnects us from the reality of ourselves and our world, the reality with which the Buddhist path is trying to reconnect us.

Thus, truly stepping into equality's expanse requires us to drop the thinking and feeling habits that separate us from what is and to courageously open to what is right here and right now. As Trungpa Rinpoche explained, "The universe is constantly trying to reach us to say something or teach something."[5] In all moments, life is inviting us to reconnect with naturalness. When we accept this invitation, daily life and everything in it becomes sacred. We honor that sacredness when we pay close attention to our direct experience and everything with which we come into contact.

PRACTICAL APPLICATION IN DAILY LIFE

Gradually, our practice and daily life begin to feel integrated, and we start to get a sense of what Milarepa described as "practice without sessions and breaks." We feel that there is more similarity between our mind in meditation practice and our mind engaged in any other activity. However, in order to accomplish this, we need the strong intention to actively integrate practice and daily life.

This section describes two different approaches for integrating practice mind in daily life and a way to frame your day in the context of "practice mind." The first approach is based on the instructions given in chapter 8 on the basic mindfulness practice of calm-abiding. In these meditations, you hold the mind to a simple point of focus, such as the breath or sensations within the body. The key objective is to keep returning the mind to its focus. Each time you are aware that you have wandered from that focus, simply notice that you have done so and return your attention to it. At points throughout the day, like when you are riding the bus or standing in line, you can do the same meditation, taking your breath or your bodily sensations—rather than your smartphone—as your focus.

Alternatively, you can make a simple task the point of focus you hold. For example, if you are washing the dishes, then do so with mindfulness. Be fully in the experience by noticing the tactile sensation of the plates and silverware in your hands, the sounds of the water splashing, and the clinking of the glasses. When your attention wanders, notice that and return your focus to the present activity. Simple tasks such as walking down the road, making a cup of tea, or showering are ideal places to start integrating mindfulness meditation into your daily life.

The second approach is to use the key points of Buddhist yogic exercise described in chapter 12 (with the exception of the Threatening Mudra, which is not suitable to use outside the practice session). Some of these exercises are related to the view of reality, such as Waves on the Ocean and Rainbow-like Reality; others are more directly concerned with connecting to the subtle body, like the Dynamic Play between Heaven and Earth, Focus on the Origin Point, and Closing the Lower Gate.

When you begin to integrate practice and daily life in this way, it is good to be specific about which focus you are working with. Choose one of the points of focus from chapter 12, and at various times during the day, recall that focus and follow the instructions for working with it for a few minutes. For example, bring to mind the view that "I" am insubstantial, like a rainbow—a dreamlike being moving within a dreamlike world—and allow that to resonate momentarily in your body-mind. Then continue with your activity. Notice the impact it has on your thoughts, feelings, and the level of tension or relaxation in your body. Making room for your felt response in your focus allows for nonconceptual direct experience to manifest, and your meditation will penetrate more deeply into your being.

It can be helpful to identify certain activities that are conducive for these moments of meditation. I particularly enjoy practicing while folding the laundry. Other times when you may want to explore integrating practice are when you first sit down at your computer, while washing the dishes, when you first get into your car before driving off, as you wait in line at the grocery store or bank, before making a phone call, when you sit down to eat or at the conclusion of your meal, or each time you return home.

As an encouragement to integrating practice mind into daily life, it can be helpful to frame your day as it begins and ends with a method for focusing your mind on practice. You can read and contemplate the sections on renunciation and compassionate bodhichitta in chapters 2 and 3 and begin your day by recalling these qualities. One way to do this (once you feel familiar with these concepts) is to recite the verses from Tilopa (page 18) and Shantideva (page 19). You can also explore your personal connection with renunciation or compassionate bodhichitta: How do you feel about them in this particular moment? How convincing or unconvincing do you find these ideas? What feels good about them? What feels more problematic about them? Which idea feels most useful to you at this point in time? This process need only take a few minutes; you are just making a little time to reconnect with them.

At the end of the day, you can close your daylong practice session by reviewing how your practice life and your emotional life were today. You are just noticing, and there is no need to add any judgment—simply know what kind of day you had. You can also appreciate any moments that seemed to go well and that you feel good about—it might even be a difficult situation you handled in a way that felt harmonious with your sense of personal integrity.

Then, if you feel so inspired, you can conclude with a dedication (for an explanation of dedicating merit, see page 24). Rather than holding on to what felt positive, share that with others. One way is to send your goodwill out to all other beings. At certain times, you may want to focus on a specific person or group of people who seem in particular need of support. Also, when you are going through a difficult time, the most important way to dedicate your practice is to yourself, to send goodwill to yourself regardless of what your experience is—anxious, angry, hopeless, or overwhelmed. You may find these words useful: "Even though I feel this anxiety/hopelessness/stress, I love and accept myself." You may also want to remind yourself of your innate worthiness by reading the words of the Buddha on page 24. When you connect with your own sense of worth and your ability to hold yourself with loving-kindness, it is much easier to believe in the worthiness of others and feel loving-kindness toward them.

If these practices ever feel too complex, you can always return to the basic foundation of practice: to develop an attitude of kindness and warmth toward yourself. So when you are confused or unsure how to practice, just come back to a sense of friendliness toward your own body and mind, your own experience. See how fully you can be with who you are in this moment and your experience in this moment, without rejecting anything about yourself.

Part Four

Exercise Instructions

12: Key Points of Buddhist Yogic Exercise

Now that the foundation for yogic exercise has been laid, we can look at some key points to apply during a practice session.

Wisdom and Compassion in Action

The basic point to remember when engaging in yogic exercise is that all Buddhist practice is about increasing our inherent qualities of wisdom and compassion. When engaging your body in any new physical activity, be cautious and proceed at a gradual, gentle pace, especially if you are not used to regular exercise. All instructions given in a book can only be general. It is essential to take these instructions and combine them with your own knowledge of your body and physical condition. This requires reexamination every practice session, as the condition of your body is continually changing. Be aware of any injuries, illnesses, or physical weaknesses that need to be taken into consideration. Throughout your sessions, be open to sensations in your body, whether the exercise feels right for you in this moment, and how far you should go with the exercise.

Listening to your own body is part of the meditational aspect of this practice; it also enhances your practice of wisdom and compassion. By taking in the information you receive from your body, you develop wisdom-awareness; by adjusting your practice so that you do not harm your body, you develop compassion. You do the same by distinguishing between pushing your body in an unhealthy, aggressive way and increasing your exertion in a healthy, positive way. Khenpo Rinpoche's instruction was to do these exercises with vigor, but each of us has to gauge what healthy vigor means for us at each given moment.

Yogic exercise is about holding our body, mind, and heart with acceptance, wisdom, and compassion. The level of vigor we use should be that which is most beneficial physically, emotionally, and mentally. In this way, we develop respect and understanding for our own bodies and what it means to inhabit a physical, subtle mind-body.

When Khenpo Rinpoche first introduced these exercises to his community, he only taught a few of them each year, so it is not necessary to do all the exercises. For beginners, it may be wise to start off gently, doing fewer exercises for a shorter period of time, and really getting to know the form and the exercise well before adding more. True yogic practice is not concerned with building up a repertoire of exercises and moving from one to the next; it focuses on deeply and fully connecting with whichever exercise we are practicing in this moment.

Khenpo Rinpoche also emphasizes that everyone's body is unique, so the exercises will look different for each of us. It is more important to connect with the fundamental meaning of each exercise rather than to try to contort your body to look like someone else's.

If you can do these exercises in bare feet, that is good, because it brings you into direct physical contact with the earth. But if you have injuries or problems with your feet or ankles, then the most skillful method is to look after them as you think best.

The following sections describe various ways of focusing during the exercises that enhance your practice of engaging wisdom when working with your body and connecting with its natural wisdom. You can pick a particular focus for each session, or you can focus in a different way for each exercise. As you become more familiar with this way of practicing, it is easier to coordinate these areas of focus with the movement, and they often arise naturally.

WAVES ON THE OCEAN

One profound way to apply the mind during any activity is to focus on the naked reality of that experience. The mind's true nature—nondual awareness, the union of luminosity-emptiness—is like a vast ocean in which thoughts and feelings are waves inseparable from that ocean. Therefore, just as waves dissolve back into the sea, you do not need to reject or subdue thoughts and feelings; you can let them naturally dissolve back into luminous awareness. Simply let your mind rest, and when an experience arises, look directly at its essence and relax.

RAINBOW-LIKE REALITY

The main point to remember about your body is that it is appearance-emptiness like a rainbow; it is purely the energy and play of luminosity-emptiness, like a body in a dream when you know you are dreaming. Recall that your body is naturally light and luminous as you practice yogic movement.

This is not only true for your own body; it is also true for the bodies of others, as well as the surrounding environment. Neither your body nor any of the outer appearances you perceive are made of the tiniest atoms, so no dividing line between these objects actually exists. As you move your body, dissolve fixation on the duality of your own body here and the surrounding environment out there. Melt into space.

DISSOLVING REFERENCE POINTS

As we work with the view described in chapter 4, we dissolve the dualistic reference points of self and other, outer and inner, mind and matter; we also challenge our habitual views of spatial location. Ordinarily, we assume that we are on the top of the planet, right side up. But directions are also dualistic concepts that do not truly exist in nondual awareness. The notion of "top" is dependent on the notion of "bottom" and vice versa. So these reference points exist only in relation to their opposite and not from their own side.

As we soften these dualistic concepts, our body and its surrounding environment reveal a gentler quality. Experience is softer because we are closer to experiencing things as they actually are. We may have sensations of being very small or very large or of vast space inside our body. These are the experiences of the subtle body, the feeling body, which is not bound by the apparent limitations of the physical world.

THE DYNAMIC PLAY BETWEEN HEAVEN AND EARTH

Another traditional way to think about the body is as an instrument of dynamic play between heaven and earth. Within each of us is an ascending energy drawing us up toward the heavens and a descending energy anchoring us on the earth. The human body and its movement are the joyful dance of this dynamic play of opposites. Rather than thinking of our movement as that of a skeletal-muscular structure, we feel it comes from allowing our body to unfold into and join these universal energies, and we simply experience them playing in space together.

To increase your awareness of this energetic pattern, begin a session by making your movements slow and rhythmic. Recall the idea of your body's movements being a dance between heaven and earth. Feel your body's sensations, and rest in whatever arises.

Wherever you hold your main focus (on your body, on various sensations, on what is arising in your mind), maintain a sense of full participation in all levels of your being, including the inner and outer ones. There is a core focus, but it is expansive enough to include all experience in its periphery.

THE DYNAMIC BODY

One way to focus is by concentrating on the movement of your body. As you tune into your body's movement, feel how it is a constantly changing and fluid field of energetic experience. Often we remove ourselves from our direct experience by engaging with conceptual chatter. We think, "I am doing well," "I am doing badly," "I am doing better than yesterday," "I don't think these exercises work," "I love this practice and should tell my friends about it." These might be thoughts you want to explore outside your practice, but during the session, just let them go. There is no need to place any judgment on yourself or what you are doing. Whenever you notice such thought patterns, return your attention to your body's movement.

SUBTLE BODY SENSATIONS IN MOVEMENT

The sensations that arise from the movements also provide a point of focus. You simply open your awareness to your bodily sensations. When conceptual chatter arises, fold it back into this awareness. The difference between focusing on the actual movement and focusing on sensations is that sensations allow you to access a more subtle experience. Concomitant images, memories, sounds, or colors may come to mind as you connect with these subtle aspects of embodied experience. If these arise for you, do not grasp them and make a big deal of them, but do not push them away either. Allow yourself to feel the experience, touch it, and then let it go.

Breathing

Specific breathing instructions are given for some of the exercises, but in general, breathe deeply, naturally, and easily. When you concentrate, you may sometimes find yourself holding your breath, which creates tension in your body. So it is always good to remember to keep breathing! Breathe deeply and fully, right down into your lower belly (for full instructions, see Lower Belly Breathing on page 113). If you feel tension in your shoulders, upper body, stomach, or lower body, then bring your breath into those areas and feel them expand and soften.

Focusing on the movement of the breath is a useful aid in meditative movement and helps you connect viscerally with your illusory, dreamlike self in this illusory, dreamlike world.

Focus on the Origin Point

The origin point is located just below your navel, deep in the center of your body. If you place your palm flat on your belly with the index finger at your navel, then the position of your little finger is roughly over the origin point. However, it is not on the surface of your belly, as the navel is, but deep in the center of your body. This is a general guide for finding this point, as it varies from person to person, depending on your proportions and the tilt of your pelvis. Most important, you find this spot by feeling into it through inner sensations rather than by measuring it with a ruler.

The origin point is considered important in many yogic traditions.[1] It can be thought of in terms of all three aspects of our being: the physical body, the subtle body, and the mind. For the physical body, the origin point is the center of gravity and literally the point from which we first developed—where our father's sperm entered the center of our mother's egg. We grew around this point, where nourishment from our mother entered and waste was expelled. The fetal position curls around this center like flower petals. Our earliest movements radiated out from the origin point and contracted back into it.

One way of understanding this point using Buddhist terminology is the principle of the mandala, which in Tibetan is *kyilkhor* (*dkyil 'khor*), literally meaning "center and surrounding." Milarepa sang of the body mandala—a sacred, whole, and complete entity but one that also has distinct parts with clear relationships to one another. One way of understanding mandala is as a microcosm of the sacred world. Similarly, one way of understanding the body is as a microcosm of the whole universe. By working with the center, the origin point, and then the entirety of our body that radiates from that point, we feel into a living, breathing, sacred mandala, and we move with that awareness.

In terms of the subtle body and mind aspects, the origin point is beyond simply being the creative source for the body; it is the source of all confusion and wisdom, the source of samsara and nirvana. Everything in experience arises from this center and dissolves back into it. It can be described as a small *bindu*, or "droplet of energy," but is capable of holding all reality; it is minutely vast. It is beyond our conceptual mind's ability to understand how this could be, but we can experience it through our yoga practice.

This small point that holds all reality is, therefore, a great center of energy in our body. When we focus mind here during movement, the subtle energy and mind gather in our body's core rather than being scattered in all directions. Gathering and concentrating ourselves in this way helps us to clarify our practice and makes it effortlessly energetic. Energy gathers at this center and also radiates out from it. This creative energy is grounded, so it flows smoothly and ceaselessly.

Throughout each session, try to maintain some awareness on the origin point. It is fine to move your attention to other parts of your body, but maintain a sense of the origin point being the source of movement and awareness. You can do this by intermittently flashing your attention on the origin point. There are further instructions in the exercise section on ways to increase your familiarity with this point and how to move from and through the origin point while lying and standing.

PRACTICING WITH VIGOR

When you move, whether slowly or quickly, generate internal vigor and strength. Move in a relaxed and natural way, but let your movements have inner strength that comes from the central core of your body. This will bring clarity to your mind and help protect you from physical injury.

Even when your body appears to be still, every part of it is actually in constant motion all the time. In its coarse state, the cells of the body are continually moving, dying and regenerating; in the subtle state, the internal winds are always flowing back and forth through their channels.

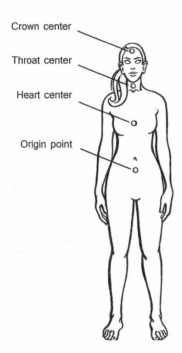

Crown center

Throat center

Heart center

Origin point

When you move your body during exercise, you can feel that you are joining your external motion with your body's continual internal movement. So rather than revving up your actions and struggling to move your body, just relax and connect with your body's natural flow of movement. Joining this natural movement and energy helps you clear away feelings of tiredness and lethargy.

At the same time, feel the vibrancy in your body by connecting with its natural alertness. Feel alive with energy. Just as with seated meditation practice, aim for being "not too tight and not too loose."

One extreme makes the body-mind dull and torpid; the other over-exerts the body-mind, depleting its core energy.

The Tibetan word that Khenpo Rinpoche uses to convey this sense of vibrancy in the body is *trimpa* (*grim pa*), meaning "drawn in." If, while sitting reading this book, you allow your body to become heavy and slack, you will feel how your energy seems to seep out. Now reverse this movement and draw your body in around the core energy centers of the origin point in your lower belly, heart center, and throat center.

You can also gently draw in the lower gate—the area of your pelvic floor (see page 104). Can you feel how the energy becomes concentrated in your body? This is a way to connect with your body's own natural reservoirs of energy.

Working with
the Threatening Mudra

A mudra that is frequently used in these exercises is called the Threatening Mudra (fig. 1). A mudra is a symbolic gesture usually made with the fingers and thumbs. In the Threatening Mudra, the middle and ring fingers of each hand are curled in and held under the thumb to make a circular shape, while the index and little fingers remain straight. This mudra is often used in ritual practice when dispelling some source of negativity and protecting what is occurring in the ritual space. It is associated with a purifying and powerful energy.

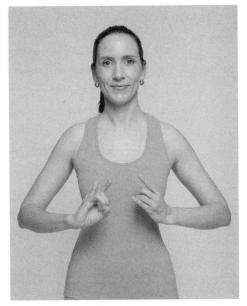

Figure 1

The fingers carry a lot of symbolic meaning in Buddhism. The middle finger is associated with purification and the ring finger with energy. Joining them with the thumb means that these principles are being engaged. This is represented in the iconography of, Manjushri, the male bodhisattva of wisdom, who is commonly depicted holding a Dharma text in his left hand between the middle and ring fingers. This symbolizes how Manjushri teaches Dharma in a completely pure way and with great energy.

As we practice with this mudra, our body-mind connects with these principles of purification and energy.

CLOSING THE LOWER GATE

The lower gate is found at the bottom of the central channel that runs from the crown of the head down through the center of the body. The center of the lower gate is positioned between the pubic bone at the front and the coccyx at the base of spine. There are different descriptions of which parts of this area are included in the lower gate; the outer boundaries are sometimes said to include the front section of the anus and the genitalia. The most important point is to develop an awareness of sensation in this area rather than trying to pinpoint the exact physical location. The lower gate is not a small point confined to a definite area, but begin your search for it by feeling the area centered between your pubic bone and coccyx. The exercise Toning the Lower Gate (see page 115) will assist you in developing familiarity with and sensory awareness of this area.

When you have some experience feeling into the lower gate and what it is like to gently squeeze it closed and let it open again after a few moments, then try using this method throughout your session. Closing the lower gate is not a tight muscular tensing but rather a subtle brightening. Initially it may feel like a muscular action, but as you progress you will develop more subtlety. It is taught that you can close the lower gate just by placing your mind's awareness there.

You may want to close the lower gate at the beginning of each exercise, as it connects you to your body's natural energy, invigorates your practice, and concentrates your mind. It can also ignite pleasant sensations in your body. Having closed the lower gate, you do not need to hold it rigidly closed. Instead, just relax. As you progress through the exercises, whenever you recall the lower gate, gently close it again—or simply focus your attention there—and continue.

Between Exercises

At the end of each exercise, it is helpful to take a brief moment to immerse yourself in the essence of your experience. Feel the sensations that arise in your body. Watch the thoughts that arise in your mind and relax in their essence—luminous spaciousness.

13: Exercises

How to Stand

MOST OF US probably feel we have a pretty good idea of how to stand. But what we are going to look at here are ways to bring more awareness to our standing posture and enhance the level of subtlety with which we engage the posture. Most of the exercises are performed standing up, so it is important that we use a posture that enhances our meditation practice.

Feet

The placement of your feet on the ground is the foundation of your standing posture and ripples up to effect the rest of your body. Spread complete wakefulness through the whole of each foot. Spread your toes out on the earth like the roots of trees. (Even if you practice indoors, the floor represents the earth element in your practice.) Imagine the main body of each foot as a rectangle, and press down into the earth through the four corners of your feet: the front of the rectangle going from the ball of the foot to the base of the little toe; the back of the rectangle being along the heel. When you press down evenly through these four points, each foot is equally balanced without rolling to the inner or outer edges. Distribute your weight evenly without leaning onto the balls of your feet or back onto your heels.

Sometimes, especially when you are focusing on learning a new exercise, you may find that your feet tense up, and your toes curl up like claws. It is helpful to notice this pattern of tension in your body and allow it to relax by melting and spreading your feet back into the earth. This may also happen in daily life; bringing awareness into your feet is a good way to reveal any tension and ground your awareness back in your body.

In terms of the subtle energies, when you press your feet down, energy rises from the centers of your feet up through your legs to the base of your spine and the bottom of the central channel. In a simple standing position, practice pressing through the four corners of your feet, lift your toes off the floor, and then gently lower them again, fanning them out fully on the floor. As you press down through your feet, feel the lift in your arches that then travels up your legs.

Knees

Keep your knees slightly bent, soft, and pliable. Even when you stand on straightening legs, never lock or hyperextend your knees; maintain a feeling of bounce in this area. This action serves two functions. First, in terms of meditation practice, the bounce in your knees helps you to connect with the fluid, dreamlike nature of experience. Second, it protects your knees and allows the energy to flow smoothly in this area. In exercises where your knees are bent and bear your weight, it is important that they be aligned in the same direction as your feet, in order to protect the joints. In other words, do not have your kneecap and your foot pointing in different directions.

Pelvis

You find balance in your pelvis by exploring the way in which your tailbone and pubic bone (at the front of the pelvis) tip. If your tailbone is overly tucked in, then the natural curve in your lumbar spine flattens out. This pattern can also lead to the chest area caving in. Conversely, if your pubic bone is overly tucked in, then your lumbar curve is exaggerated and your bottom sticks out. For good balance, aim to have your tailbone and pubic bone dropping evenly and curving toward each other. Richard Freeman, a great American yoga scholar and teacher, speaks of encouraging the tailbone and pubic bone to kiss. They lean in to one another with equal attraction.

We look for the same equilibrium in the sides of the body between the left and right hips. Try to sense whether one hip drops lower than the other, and work toward evening them out.

When your pelvis is balanced in this way, your lower back is protected and a stable foundation is created for your upper back. This is particularly important in exercises where your knees are bent and weight-bearing, such as Shooting Arrow Yoga (page 141) and Indestructible Vajra Posture (page 148), where people sometimes stick their bottom out, creating tension and discomfort in their lower back.

Heart and Shoulders

When your lower body is aligned correctly, your upper body has a stable foundation and can unfurl upward in space, like the trunk and branches of a tree that has solid roots in the earth. Your heart is like a flower, blossoming in all directions and filling the back of your body as much as the front. Your shoulders support the opening of your heart; when they are firmly rooted, with the scapulae (shoulder blades) flowing smoothly down the back of your body, your heart naturally becomes buoyant.

When moving your arms, you may tend to lift your shoulders up and out of the shoulder girdle. Doing this creates strain in the shoulder and neck area. To maintain the integrity of your shoulder joints, try to refrain from lifting your upper arms out of the shoulder sockets, even when you lift or stretch your arms out in exercises such as Shooting Arrow Yoga (page 141) and the Four-Limb Exercise (page 133).

A simple exercise to illustrate this is to reach your right arm out and up, like you are reaching for an apple from a tree that is in front of you and slightly to the right. Allow your arm to lift out of the shoulder joint and the scapula to slide up with your arm. Keeping your arm in this position, firmly draw the scapula down your back and your upper arm into the shoulder socket. This second position is how you maintain the integrity of your shoulder joints in these exercises. Even as you keep this placement, try to allow your shoulders and upper arms to remain as soft and fluid as possible.

Head and Eyes

By patterning your heart and shoulders correctly, you give your head a supportive foundation that allows it to float effortlessly at the top of your spine. Your jaw and earlobes relax downward and allow your soft palate to release. The soft palate rises upward, like the bright peak of a snow mountain, toward the crown of your head. Your gaze is soft but wakeful.

DISPELLING THE STALE BREATH

Begin in standing posture with your arms at your sides. Breathe in through your nose slowly and deeply into your lower belly. Imagine your lower belly as a ball that expands in all directions as you inhale rather than just out in front. As you breathe in, your hands make fists around your thumbs, which are placed at the base of your ring fingers (fig. 2). Once you have completed an inhalation, hold the breath for a few seconds in a ball below your navel (fig. 3).

Exhale gently through your nostrils. At the end of the exhalation, forcefully push out all of the air from your belly up and spread out your palms and fingers. To exhale fully, pull your lower belly in toward your spine in a firm but gentle contraction. You can also gently squeeze the lower gate to complete the exhalation (fig. 4).

Repeat this three times: first exhale all sickness, then all negativity, and finally all mental fabrications. The Tibetan word for negativity is *don* (*gdon*), which is often used to refer to malevolent forces and various types of demons. In this context, we can understand these malevolent forces to be difficult states of mind such as fear, depression, and anxiety. "Mental fabrications" refer to the complex web of ideas that we overlay on our experience of simple and direct reality—they are all the things mind makes up about itself, its world, and its experience.

At the conclusion of the third exhalation, take a moment to rest in simple, naked awareness. This is the nondual, unborn state, beyond something to be purified and someone doing the purification. By doing this, you combine the skillful means of purifying sickness, negativity, and mental fabrications with the true nature of reality that is beyond such concepts. You unite appearances (the apparent display of such things as sickness and negativity) with emptiness (the lack of solidity in these appearances).

Dispelling the Stale Breath can be done at the beginning of all your meditation practice sessions. It is also good to do when you first wake up in the morning or anytime you want to relax and clear your mind. It can be performed seated, standing, or even lying down.

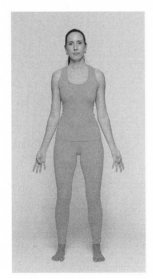
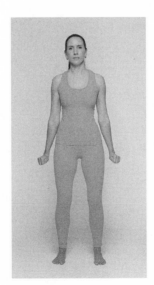
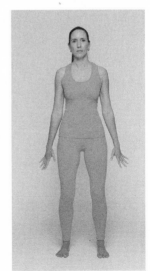

Figure 2   *Figure 3*   *Figure 4*

PREPARATORY EXERCISES

To prepare your body for the session, start by stimulating its subtle channels by tapping around it lightly. You can use a flat palm or a loosely held fist with your thumb outside your fingers.

Begin tapping on the inside of your upper left arm and down

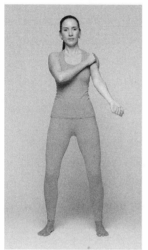

Figure 5

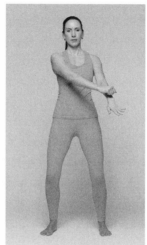

Figure 6

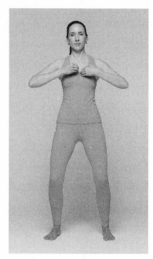

Figure 7

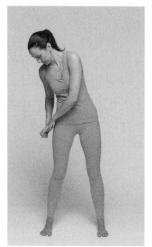

Figure 8

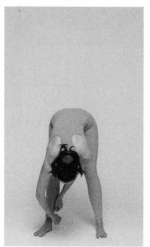

Figure 9

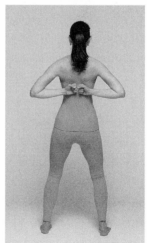

Figure 10

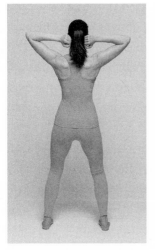
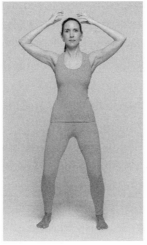
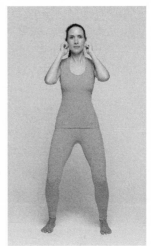

Figure 11   Figure 12   Figure 13

your wrist (fig. 5). Then turn your left arm and tap up the outside (fig. 6). Do the same on your right arm. Then tap across your upper chest from left to right—you may want to just use your fingertips (fig. 7). Then do your legs, begin with both hands on the outside of your upper right leg, tapping all the way down to your ankle (fig. 8). Then tap up your inner right leg (fig. 9). Repeat on your left leg.

Now place the backs of your fists on either side of your spine, as high up your back as you can reach (fig. 10). Massage the sides of your spine with your fists. Gradually work down your back to your buttocks.

Next, lightly tap the neck muscles on either side of your spine (fig. 11). Tap your head with your fingertips; you can include your forehead and cheeks (fig. 12). Conclude by massaging your ears between your thumbs and the base of your index fingers, from the tops of your ears down to the bottom of the earlobes (fig. 13).

Lower Belly Breathing

This exercise helps you to develop deep breathing and brings awareness down into your lower belly.

Lie on your back with your knees bent and your feet flat on the floor. If the floor is hard, you may wish to put a yoga mat or blanket beneath you. You can either place your hands with palms down on your lower belly or alongside you on the floor with the palms up. Allow the natural curves in your spine and neck to remain; try to have your face parallel with the ground, without tucking your chin in or sticking it up in the air.

On the inhalation, focus on bringing the breath down toward the origin point so that it fills your lower belly; you will feel your stomach expand. Your pelvis will naturally tilt to accommodate the breath, increasing your lumbar curve. The space between your lower back and the floor will increase (fig. 14).

On the exhalation, focus on completely emptying your lower belly. To accomplish this, gently draw your lower stomach in toward your spine. Try to feel into the more subtle sensations of your body, especially the motion coming from the energetic sheath of your stomach. As your stomach empties, your tailbone will tilt upward and the space between your lower back and the floor will decrease. As you become familiar with this movement, you can also complete the exhalation by closing the lower gate (fig. 15).

Do at least twenty-one cycles of breath in this position. Once you find it easy to connect with breathing into your lower belly in the movement exercises, you may not need to perform this exercise in every practice session.

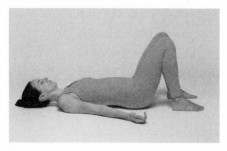

Figure 14

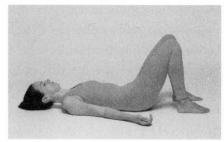

Figure 15

This exercise can be very helpful when you are feeling anxious and ungrounded. You can also practice lower belly breathing while seated or in Horse Posture (see page 131). Try focusing on the breath coming down evenly into your belly. A common tendency is to allow the front of the belly to soften and expand while the back body is stiff and constricted. Here, as you breathe down into your belly, try to soften and expand your lower back area as well as the front of your belly, as though a ball is being evenly inflated in your lower belly. Starting any seated meditation practice with a few rounds of lower belly breathing grounds you in your body, laying a good foundation for practice.

Toning the Lower Gate

This exercise helps you develop familiarity with the lower gate. Start by lying on your back (again if you are on a hard surface, you may wish to place a blanket or yoga mat beneath you). Align your head evenly with the floor, with your chin neither poking up nor tucked in. Then bring your knees up toward your body and hold them with your arms. Strongly draw each knee toward the corresponding armpit. If you are flexible or have long arms, you can use your forearms rather than your hands.

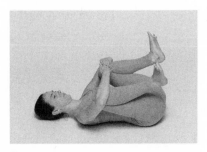

Figure 16

As you bring your knees in, you will feel your tailbone lift off the ground and curl inward. Try to tip your pubic bone down to kiss your tailbone. You will be working with opposing patterns—as you pull your pubic bone downward, you will have to hold your knees firmly to keep your tailbone lifting. The pelvic floor muscles work hard in this position, which creates a lot of sensation in the area of the lower gate. The lower gate brightens and tones.

Once sensation has arisen in this area, hold the position for a few moments and keep your awareness focused on your pelvic floor.

Then release your feet down to the ground and maintain your attention on the sensations. Repeat a few times so you feel you have really connected with this area. At the end of the repetitions, lie flat on the floor and allow your awareness to maintain a central focus on the lower gate area as well as some peripheral awareness of your whole body.

Six-Limb Radiation from the Origin Point (on the Floor)

One of the central focal points in this practice is the origin point. The lower belly breathing exercise you just did helps you bring your breath—and thus also awareness—down into your lower belly. In this exercise, you will begin working with movement that radiates from and then contracts back into this center.

Lie on your back on the floor, and bring your awareness into the origin point at the center of your lower belly. Exhale and curl

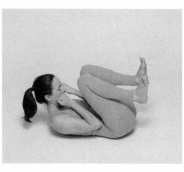

your whole body—including your hands, head, and feet—up and around this point (fig. 17). On the inhalation, gradually spread the breath so that it fills your whole body evenly, like blowing up a balloon. As the breath spreads, so do your six limbs: your arms, legs, head, and tailbone. Open and stretch out fully across the floor, like a starfish uncurling on the bottom of the sea

Figure 17

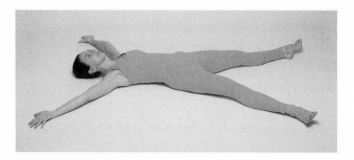

Figure 18

(fig. 18). On your next exhalation, draw back into the curled-up position.

As you repeat these movements that are synchronized with your breath, feel your body's fluidity and the rhythm this movement creates in your body, like the ebb and flow of the sea. The movement expands from and contracts to the origin point evenly. Maintain a focus on your core center at the origin point while feeling the harmony in this movement between your core and the periphery of your limbs. Feel how your limbs organize themselves and communicate with each other via the origin point. This exercise is called "six-limb" because the head and tailbone are included with the legs and arms. Remember to curl and uncurl them as well. It is important to connect with how your body arranges itself through the origin point and the sensation of bodily wholeness and harmony during all the following exercises.

MAIN EXERCISES

Dance of the Warriors

Stand with your legs in a fairly wide stance, a little less than one leg's length apart (you can bring them a little closer if necessary). Turn your feet out slightly, and press evenly through all four corners of each foot. Hold your hands in the Threatening Mudra (page 103). Your body faces forward at the beginning, but as you move through the exercise, your upper body will follow the movement of your arms to each side.

To begin, just try the leg movement while holding your hands on your hips. Your legs simply lunge from one side to the other: first your weight is over your left leg, which bends while your right leg straightens; then you shift your weight over to your right leg, which bends while your left leg straightens. Try to keep the movement fluid as you shift from side to side. As the bent leg is weight-bearing, make sure that the knee bends out in the same direction as the foot.

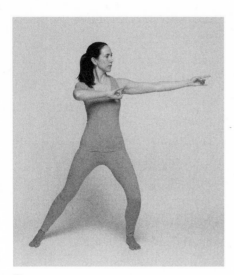

Figure 19

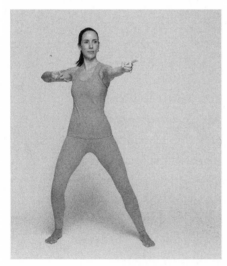

Figure 20

Now try adding the arms and hands in Threatening Mudra (fig. 19). Start by bending and leaning on your left leg while keeping your right leg straight. Hold your left arm straight out at shoulder-height with your palm facing out and the index finger uppermost. Bend your right arm in with your hand held in front of your left shoulder, your palm facing out with the little finger uppermost. Then draw your straightened left arm around in a semicircle across to your right side (fig. 20). Feel as though you have a pen in your hand and the paper is a little in front of you, so you need to stretch your arm out, while keeping your body erect and your upper arm firmly in the shoulder socket with the scapula gliding down your back. This creates a wonderful stretch through the whole length of your arm.

As your left arm finishes the arc of the semicircle, bend it so that your left hand comes level to your right shoulder; turn your hand over so that the little finger is uppermost, the thumb is lowest, and the palm faces away from you. Simultaneously, reach your right arm straight out to the right with the index finger uppermost, the little finger lowest, and the palm facing out. As your arms complete these movements, move your legs from lunging to the left to lunging to the right. Your left and right arms are now in the starting position, but you are facing the opposite direction (fig. 21).

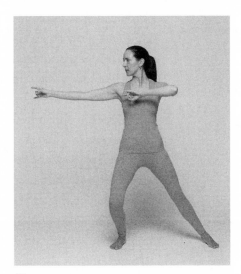

Figure 21

Either allow your eyes and head to follow the movement of your arms, or simply face forward and find a spot on the ground a few feet in front of you on which to gently rest your gaze. Feel that your arms and legs are full of energy, and there is an ease and grace in your body. Work on creating a smooth transition from side to side. Do not pause or hold the movement as you reach one side; simply and smoothly move toward the other side again, so your body is in continuous movement.

See if you can feel the stretch in the straight arm and straightening leg while simultaneously holding awareness in your origin point. Feel how your whole body moves from this point, so your core is strongly aligned yet your body is stretching at the same time. Do not let your shoulders lift toward your ears, and do not tip your body over to the left or right as you move, but remain upright.

Generally, it is best to begin this exercise slowly until you have a smooth flow of movement. Then you can play with the speed, building up to a faster pace if you can retain your meditative awareness.

As you speed up, the movement in your legs decreases. Rather than lunging from side to side, bounce on your knees with your arms in more rapid motion. There is a slight swing from side to side. Your arms come in front of your body, and your hands and forearms spin from your elbows. To accomplish this, you will need to keep your arms relaxed and loose; keep the core of your body strong and steady. With your eyes, keep a soft but steady gaze directed a few feet in front of you.

You can speed up and slow down a few times in one practice. At the end, slow down and move toward stillness. Once you have stopped moving your legs and arms, just wiggle your toes and your fingers like leaves on a tree blowing in the wind. Then bring your body to complete stillness and feel the sensations in it. Notice what your body feels like now, in this moment.

This exercise is good for loosening up your entire body and infusing it with spacious and relaxed awareness. If you are just beginning to work with all the various points of attention—the closing of the lower gate, focusing on the origin point, and the view of the body's dreamlike and illusory nature—concentrating on this one exercise can help you coordinate these elements.

This exercise is also useful when you are feeling physically unwell or are dealing with difficult emotions. As you move, focus your mind on the places in your body that are painful, sick, or tense. This helps in the healing process. Or you can simply focus on the fluidity of the body-mind and increase your overall mental relaxation.

Three-Limb Exercise

In this exercise, you balance on one leg. If you are prone to falling or easily become dizzy, you can use a wall to stabilize yourself. If you are simply a little wobbly and need more practice balancing, it is best to forgo a support so that your body learns how to balance. For most of us, the fear of falling in this exercise is not a fear of actual physical harm; it is a fear of failure, appearing foolish, or something equally unpleasant. Sometimes the best way to practice is to give ourselves permission to look a bit messy and to be playful. We can remind ourselves that even if we appear to "fail," this does not damage our innate worth. Then we connect with the wisdom of wobbling a little, of being a bit of a fool—we learn that we survive such moments and may even come to enjoy them!

When you lose your balance, simply put your foot down and then bring it up again—your body will gradually learn to balance.

Maintaining a fixed eye gaze helps with balance, so choose a point on the floor or wall, no higher than your eyes, on which to focus and maintain your gaze on this point. You can also imagine that your supporting foot is spreading across the ground and growing roots down into the earth. Feel your weight being sent down into the earth; this helps to create a stable foundation.

Start by trying the leg movement. From a simple standing position, with your hands on your hips, bring your weight into your left foot. Keep your left knee slightly bent. Try to maintain the integrity of your hip joint; as your weight moves into your left leg, do not allow your left hip to jut out to the left, but keep your hips evenly aligned. Lift your right leg, with the knee bent, positioned diagonally out to the front and right. Do not bring your knee higher than your hip. Circle your ankle and knee inward. As the circle is completed, flick your leg out with the foot flexed and toes pointing upward—like kicking a soccer ball. Try this movement a few times on each side while keeping your hands on your hips, and then try the arm movement.

Your arms move in a similar way. Extend them out to the sides at shoulder-height. Hold your hands in Threatening Mudra. Bend from your elbows and circle your wrists and forearms up and inward, then forcefully flick your arms out in a strong movement. Your arms finish straight out to the sides with your hands pulled back from your wrists a little so that the fingers are pointing up to the sky and the palms face out. Try the movements with your hands and arms a few times until they feel familiar.

Now try synchronizing all the movements (fig. 22). As your lifted foot and

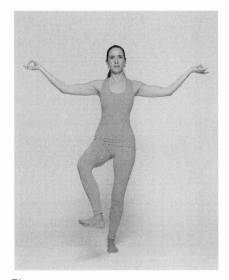

Figure 22

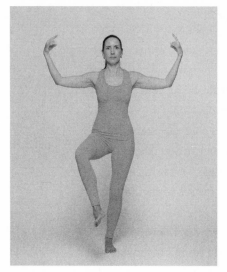

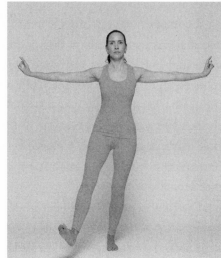

Figure 23   Figure 24

calf circle inward, so do your wrists and arms (fig. 23). Then all three limbs strongly flick outward (fig. 24). Leave a slight pause and then repeat the movements. Start with twenty-one repetitions on each leg.

Keep your lifted thigh and upper arms strongly engaged to protect your joints in the final flicking motion. Even though your arms and legs flick outward, there is a simultaneous sensation of energy drawing into your core body. You should feel a good stretch and extension through your arms and legs, but do not overextend your elbows or knees.

These movements help to straighten the channels through which the body's subtle inner winds flow. Various elements of life can cause these channels to contract and knot, preventing the winds from flowing smoothly. This leads to various disturbances of the mind and heart and can also lead to physical problems. Stretching out these channels allows the inner winds to flow smoothly again.

Rotation Series

This is a series of rotations around points in the central channel. The movements are initiated from deep inside your body, stretching and energizing the whole area. These rotations help to release any knotted or blocked energy in your body's core. Keep the motion fluid and relaxed. At the conclusion of each of these exercises, spread any warmth, ease, or relaxation that has arisen throughout your entire body.

When you rotate your torso, it is important to create space in your spine so that the vertebrae do not crunch into one another. To create this space, start by elongating your spine. Begin in a simple standing posture with your feet hip-width apart, then raise your heels a few inches off the floor. While maintaining the height of your head and heart, slowly extend your heels back down to the earth. When you lift your heels, you can place your hand on top of your head. As your heels descend, keep your hand at its original height and reach your head up toward your hand. Sense the elongation in your spine. Start all of these rotations from that place (fig. 25).

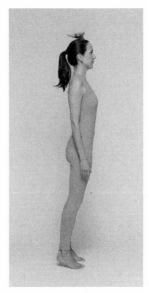

Figure 25

Rotate the Origin Point

In standing posture, with your feet hip-width apart, knees slightly bent, and your hands resting gently on your hips, bring your attention down into the origin point; feel into any sensations in this area. Begin rotating around this center, ensuring that the movement is initiated from this core rather than being a grosser movement of your physical body (fig. 26).

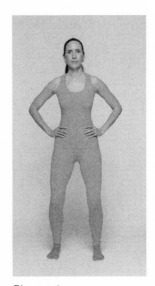

Figure 26

To feel into the subtlety of this movement, keep it small, so that it would be barely perceptible to an outside observer. Gradually increase the movement to include rotation of your hips, but keep the focus deep in the core of your body. Keep your knees soft and flexible to allow for the movement, but move only your hip area with intention. Circle clockwise several times and then counterclockwise. When you have rotated a few times in each direction, move into stillness. Take a moment to observe any sensations in your lower belly or your entire body.

Rotate the Heart Center

Bring your awareness to your heart center and feel into any sensations there. We often hold a lot of emotional energy in our heart center, so you may find some intense sensations. Gently circle your shoulders back one at a time, allowing space and sensitivity for your emotional experience (figs. 27 and 28). Once you have started moving, you may find that the sensations relax and become more spacious, in which case, you can increase the movement. But keep the movement small and gentle if that feels more appropriate.

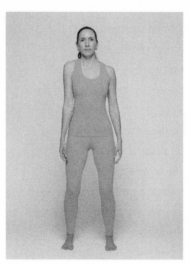
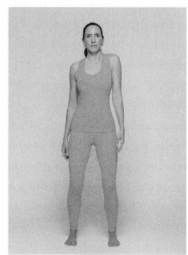

Figure 27   *Figure 28*

Simply circle your shoulders backward, alternating right and left, with your arms at your sides. As in the previous exercise, the movement is initiated from the core of your body, from your heart center. After rotating backward several times, reverse the movement and rotate your shoulders forward several times. Then move into stillness and notice what your heart's sensations feel like now.

Rotate the Throat Center

Bring awareness to your throat center, deep in the center of your throat (you will probably feel this somewhere in the area between your Adam's apple and the two knobs of the collarbones at the base of your neck). With your arms relaxed at your sides, feel that your neck is elongated.

Roll your head three times in each direction. If you have had a neck injury or feel any tension or discomfort in your neck, simply lean your head forward and slowly and gently move it in semicircles between your shoulders or in whatever smaller way feels appropriate for you. Be sure to listen to your body and only do what feels right. Whatever movement you choose, initiate it from your throat center and maintain awareness there. Keep your eyes open during all these rotation exercises.

Drop the Crown Center

Bring your awareness to the crown center at the top of your head. With relaxed shoulders and neck, let your head drop heavily forward so that your chin reaches toward your lower neck (fig. 29). Do this a few times, maintaining your focus at your crown.

Wet Wooly Sheep Shake Out

In this exercise, we loosen the body and shake every part of it out. This is a wonderful way to release tension, contraction, and stagnation and to reboot

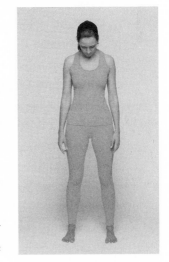

Figure 29

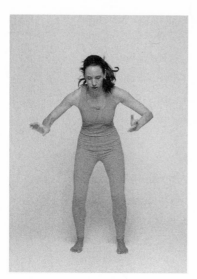

Figure 30

the body-mind. It follows an instinctual action in both humans and animals—when we remember something bad, we physically shudder in order to shake off any unpleasant associations we have with that image.

Stand with your feet about hip-width apart and your knees slightly bent. Keep your lower body firmly grounded but still flexible, your arms relaxed at your sides. Inhale, and then as you exhale, shake out your upper body: your head, cheeks, and lips; shoulders, arms, and hands (fig. 30). Let everything be loose and easily shaken. Repeat the shake out a few times, synchronizing it with the breath by first breathing in and then shaking out on the exhalation. Once you have shaken out your upper body, remain in stillness momentarily and feel your bodily sensations.

Then shake out your hips, thighs, and stomach—jiggle everything that can be jiggled from your upper stomach through your thighs.

Finally, shake your legs out one at a time, just loosely kicking them out in front of you. This is not a strong, forceful kick as in the Three-Limb Exercise, but a simple, loose kick that allows your thigh, knee, calf, ankle, foot, and toes to shake around and release.

This is a wonderful exercise to engage in spontaneously anytime you need a reboot. It can also be modified to fit any situation. For example, while still sitting at your computer, you can gently shake out your head and upper body and see how that makes you feel. While seated, you can also wiggle your bottom to loosen up your hip, stomach, and thigh areas. It is beneficial to practice this exercise when you are stressed or upset, but it is also useful to do it periodically without a particular impetus, especially if your days are quite sedentary.

Wrist and Ankle Rotations

Rotating your wrists and ankles is important in keeping your body loose and flexible, especially if you spend a lot of time using a computer keyboard.

Hold your hands in prayer position, level with your chest (fig. 31). Rotate your hands forward and down from the wrists, then back and inward so that your fingertips draw the outer circumference of a circle (fig. 32). Keep your wrists as close to each other as possible so that you feel a good stretch as you turn them. Circle forward ten times and then back ten times.

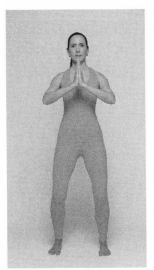

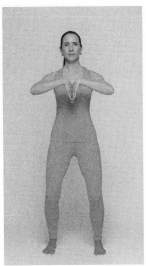

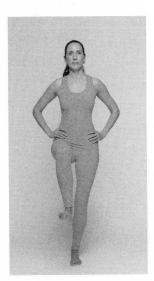

Figure 31   Figure 32   Figure 33

Stand on your left leg with your hands on your hips. Raise your right leg so that your thigh is parallel with the floor. Rotate your right ankle ten times in each direction, making as big a circle as possible, and then repeat the exercise on your left leg (fig. 33).

Vertical Wheel of Fire

In ancient India, wandering entertainers would twirl a lit torch in front of them, creating the illusion of an unbroken wheel of fire. That is where the name of this exercise comes from; you are going to be making a continuous circular motion with your hands that simulates the circular movement of that torch.

Begin by standing with your legs a little wider than your hips, your feet roughly parallel and rooting into the ground, and your pelvis aligned—dropping your tailbone and pubic bone equally so that your bottom is not sticking out or overly tucked in. Allow your knees to bend softly.

Hold your hands in Threatening Mudra in front of you with the palms facing each other about a foot apart and level with your head. Keeping your hands in this position, move them both in a circular motion, as though your hands are drawing circles in the space

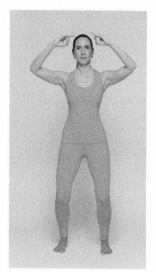
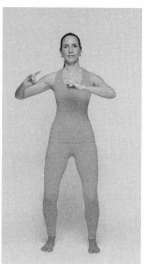
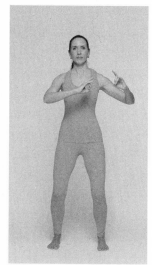

Figure 34   Figure 35   Figure 36

in front of you. Rotate both hands in the same direction so that they stay roughly the same distance from each other as they move around. Synchronize the bending of your knees with the circling of your hands: as your arms move down to the bottom half of the circle, bend your knees; as they come up the circle and return level with your head, straighten your legs (but do not lock your knees).

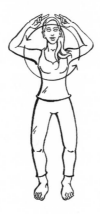

As you move, focus on a circle rotating around the origin point in your lower belly, also on the same upright plane as the circles that your hands are drawing. In Tibetan, this movement is called *pokhor* (*sbo 'khor*), literally "belly circle." The circling action of the arms and stomach area are all initiated from this circling in the lower belly.

Start circling slowly, gradually building up the speed and force of the exercise. After going in one direction for awhile, decrease the vigor, change direction, and repeat. You can change direction a few times in a session. As you move more quickly, you may find your clarity increases. When you rest in that clarity without getting attached to it, identifying with it, or defining it as anything, you are resting in clarity-emptiness inseparable. As you decrease the force, relax your mind, and let it rest at ease.

Make sure to bend your knees so that you include your whole

body in the movement. Keep in mind the image of circling. Focus on the sensations within your body, and as you move into stillness at the conclusion of this exercise, just rest in whatever sensations have arisen in your body. Khenpo Rinpoche calls this resting in the luminosity of our sensations the "delight of the yogis and yoginis."

This exercise can help resolve sicknesses in your digestive system and the lower part of your body.

Horizontal Wheel of Fire

This exercise is similar to the previous one except that all the circles are made on a horizontal plane, like stirring a giant pot with two spoons. Start with your hands in Threatening Mudra, and hold them about a foot apart out in front of your belly. They should mirror each other—the outstretched fingers point to their counterpart on the opposite hand, the little fingers are lowest, and the thumbs and index fingers are uppermost (as though the curled-in fingers were holding the stirring spoons). The circles your hands make in this position are parallel to the ground. The origin point also circles

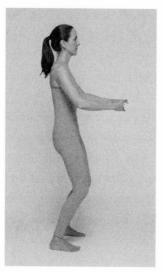
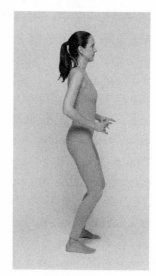

Figure 37   *Figure 38*

on the horizontal plane. As your hands circle in toward your belly, your abdomen circles back, away from your hands. As your hands circle away from your body, your belly circles forward. So the distance between your hands and belly remains roughly the same throughout the movement.

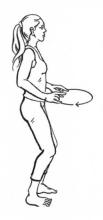

As in the previous exercise, circle in one direction and then switch. You can also gradually increase the speed and then decrease it.

Horse and Squat Postures

These two postures are beneficial in themselves and also help in the Four-Limb Exercise that follows. The first is Horse Posture, which strengthens your thighs and cultivates a sense of confidence and grounding in the body-mind (fig. 39). Stand with your feet a little wider than your hips; bend your knees (you can play with how much you bend, depending on how hard you want to work your thigh muscles). Allow your hands to either hang at your sides or rest on your thighs; keep your pelvis aligned and your back upright. Allow your scapulae to flow down to the earth and your heart and head to float. Release your soft palate with the syllable AH. Allow your earlobes and jaw to let go as your soft palate brightens and lifts toward your crown.

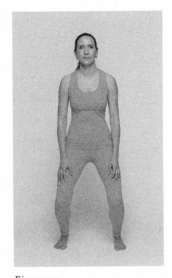

Figure 39

You can hold this posture and practice Lower Belly Breathing (described on page 113). Bring the breath down to the origin point; allow your belly to soften and expand on the inhalation and to contract gently on the exhalation. You can place your hands, one above the other, over the origin point to help you focus on that area. This is a wonderful standing meditation practice, and if you have trouble sitting for long periods in practice sessions, you can alternate sitting meditation with this standing method.

People commonly squatted before sitting in chairs became so prevalent, and many traditional cultures still use this posture when people gather together. Children naturally assume this posture as they play or investigate the miracles of a bug trundling about the garden. There is a level of comfort in this posture that may partly come from its similarity to the fetal position. It feels natural and in tune with the childlike awareness that is endlessly curious and joyful. You can nestle into this posture and feel contained and whole. Energetically, this posture is very grounding, and once you have become comfortable in it, it can be deeply relaxing.

Stand with your feet hip distance apart, and bend your knees as low as you comfortably can without having them collapse in toward each other. Try to keep the upper body in an upright plane. Ensure that your knees are tracking in the exact direction of your feet and that your feet are not rolling onto their inner arch or outer edge. To protect your joints, it is more important that your alignment is correct and you stay higher than that you bend lower but lose the integrity of the pose. This way you will strengthen your muscles and train them to maintain correct alignment, so that over time you will be able to go lower.

If you are in the full squat (bending your knees fully and bringing your bottom down behind your heels, while keeping your heels on the ground), you can alternate between holding your legs and feet together with your arms around the outside of your legs (fig. 40) and parting your feet and legs while bringing your arms inside your legs (fig. 41). When your legs are together, try to keep your heels on the ground and do not rock too far forward, keeping your weight balanced. You will feel the muscles on the outer edges of your shins activate and your feet engage. When your feet are apart, you can lean your body a little farther forward and bring your outer upper arms inside your knees with your hands in front of you in prayer position. This will give you an additional stretch in your lower back. You can also push out with your upper arms while simultaneously pressing in with your knees, creating more stretch and strengthening the muscles.

If you cannot do a full squat, then you can work your way into it from Horse Posture. Once you feel comfortable holding Horse Posture for a few minutes, you can gradually work on bringing your legs a little closer and bending lower, until one day you may comfortably squat down.

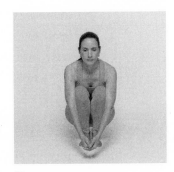

Figure 40

Four-Limb Exercise

Stand with your feet slightly wider than your hips, and crouch down as far as your knees and back will allow (fig. 41). If you cannot go very low, it will look more like Horse Posture (page 131), which is fine. Place your thumbs at the base of each ring finger and draw your hands into fists by curling your fingers around your thumbs, as in Dispelling the Stale Breath (page 110). Bring your arms between your knees, drawing your body into a gentle ball.

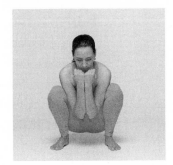

Figure 41

Next, rise up strongly, with your feet pressing firmly into the ground and extend your arms upward in a V-shape with your hands outstretched (fig. 42). Look out and up. As you rise, exhale fully from the bottom of your belly through your mouth. As you exhale, make an aspirated hah sound. Keep your feet on the floor throughout this exercise, with your heels firmly grounded, if possible, even in the crouched position. Keep your knees aligned in the direction of your feet, especially as you bend down. Your

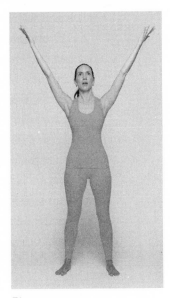

Figure 42

feet should be turned outward very slightly and a little more than a foot apart so that you can comfortably come down with your arms inside the legs. Keep repeating these movements: inhale each time you come down, and forcefully exhale as you rise. Do this ten or twenty times, or more if you feel like it.

There is a traditional visualization that goes with this exercise. In the sky in front of you is a white syllable HA, which you can visualize in Tibetan, English, or whatever alphabet you are most familiar with. In your heart center, facing outward, is another HA, but this one is dark blue or black. Visualize that the HA in your heart center is full of any negative feelings you have—stress, anger, anxiety, depression, and tension. As you exhale, some of this negativity is sent up to the white HA. As you repeat the exercise, the white HA in the sky gradually darkens, and the dark HA in your heart gradually lightens. Eventually, the HA in the sky is completely dark, and the HA in your heart is completely white—all the negative feelings from your body-mind have been sent up to the HA in the sky. At the completion of the exercise, dissolve both HAS into empty space. Take a few minutes to rest your mind in space, free from any reference point.

This exercise was traditionally used in Tibet to help with anxiety disorders. It was found to be particularly effective for those who studied a lot or practiced a lot of meditation and became contracted or tight, particularly in the heart. Khenpo Rinpoche has recommended that some people who suffer from anxiety disorders, stress, or anger issues concentrate mainly on this exercise until they experience some relief.

Garuda Posture

In legend, the *garuda* (a mythical birdlike creature often depicted with a human body) is said to have a vast wingspan that can block out the sun and create hurricanelike winds when flapped. Position your legs and feet in Horse Posture, with your arms at your sides.

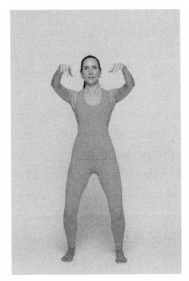
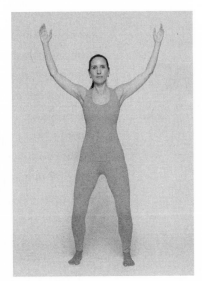

Figure 43   Figure 44

Imagine that your arms are giant wings. Lift them up in front of you and then gently circle them backward and down to make a full circle. Do this slowly and rhythmically rather than swinging them. After circling them backward, you can also circle them forward.

During this exercise, maintain a panoramic awareness that stretches out in all directions. Focus your awareness behind, above, and below you, not just out in front. Repeat this exercise seven or twenty-one times in each direction, or you can do more if you feel like it. This is a great exercise to do outdoors, particularly in a place that has an expansive view. If you are indoors, simply recall a sense of vast spaciousness.

Standing Radiation from the Origin Point

This is a standing balance version of the floor exercise Six-Limb Radiation from the Origin Point and uses the same principles of movement.

From a simple standing position, bring your weight into your left leg, root your left foot firmly down into the floor, and establish a

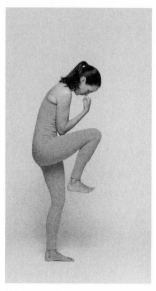

Figure 45

point for your gaze out in front of you and slightly down to help you balance. On an inhalation, raise your right knee, and on the exhalation draw in your right leg and foot while simultaneously curling your entire upper body and arms around the origin point, fisting your hands around your thumbs (fig. 45). On the next inhalation, evenly expand your body, arms, hands, leg, foot, and toes outward in a smooth flowing movement. Extend your right leg behind you and allow your toes to touch the floor (fig. 46). On the next exhalation, draw everything back in again around the origin point. Do ten or twenty repetitions with each leg.

When you feel comfortable balancing in this exercise, you can do the same initial movement, but instead of allowing your foot to touch the

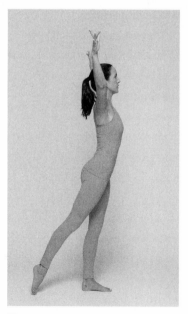

Figure 46

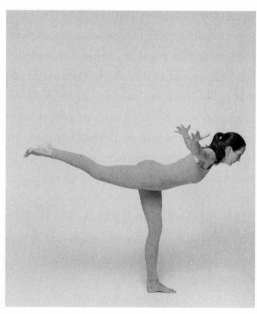

Figure 47

ground on the inhalation, bring your leg straight out behind you and lean forward into a balance. Allow your arms to stretch out to either side (fig. 47).

As you repeat these movements synchronized with your breath, feel your body's fluidity and the rhythm the movements create in your body, like the ebb and flow of the sea. The movement should expand evenly throughout your body and then contract just as evenly back to the origin point. Maintain a focus on your core center at the origin point, but feel the harmony in this movement between your core and your limbs. Feel how your limbs organize themselves and communicate with each other via your core.

Dance of the Warrior Laughing at Appearances

Stand with your feet a little less than one leg's length apart and your hands in Threatening Mudra at your sides. As you turn to the left, bend your left knee a little and straighten the right so that most of your weight is on your left foot. Your right heel can come off the ground a bit if this helps you in the turning motion. Bring your right arm across your body, and flick it out to the left; flick your left arm straight out behind you, so together they make a straight diagonal line. As you flick your arms, make sure that your upper arm and shoulder muscles are strongly engaged; keep your upper arms in the shoulder joints. Stay grounded in your body and keep it upright; do not lean out toward the front arm. Make sure that your feet and legs are not rigid; keep them flexible, with plenty of bounce (fig. 48).

Look out and up in the direction of your right hand, which is pointing up to space. Do the same movement to the other side and then keep switching from side to side. As you come through center, draw your arms in (fig. 49) and then flick them out as you move to the opposite side (fig. 50). As you twist in the first direction, cry, "HA HA"; as you twist in the opposite direction, cry, "HEE HEE." This is the sound of laughter. As you progress with the exercise, you can gradually speed up the pace and then slow it down; you

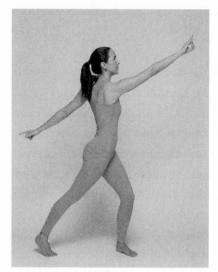

Figure 48

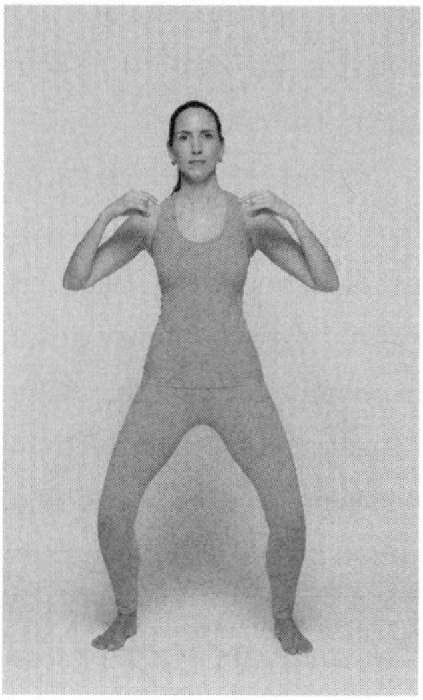

Figure 49

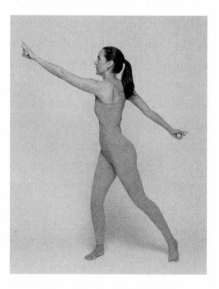

Figure 50

can alter the speed a few times in one session. At the end, gradually settle into stillness.

The following verse by Khenpo Rinpoche goes well with this exercise:

Look at appearance—emptiness forms,
Listen to sound and emptiness sounds,
Rest in mind's nature, clarity-emptiness,
And when your thoughts free themselves,
Laugh, oh laugh, "HA HA! HEE HEE!"[1]

As we make the sounds of laughter, we know that all the appearances of forms that seem to cause us so many problems are unreal, merely appearance-emptiness. We recognize how we get lost in anger, jealousy, anxiety, or desire because we take these appearances so seriously; we fixate on them as solid entities. The same is true for the sounds we hear. When we realize this and rest in mind's nature (clarity-emptiness), our difficult thoughts self-liberate because they have no fuel to maintain them. At that point, the only suitable expression is to laugh: HA HA! HEE HEE!

Warrior Lunge

Stand with your feet nearly one leg's length apart, with your feet turned out slightly and your hands in Threatening Mudra, tucked

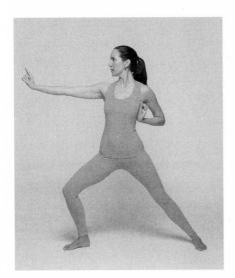

Figure 51

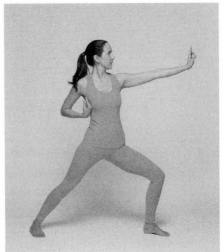

Figure 52

under your armpits. Your legs lunge from side to side in this exercise but your torso faces forward. Begin by lunging right and strongly extend your right hand out from under your armpit by dragging the back of your hand down the side of your body and firmly out, giving your side a good massage—the movement is like striking a match. As your right arm straightens to the side, point the fingers upward; look toward your fingertips and the space beyond. Your left hand remains curled under your left armpit. Then lunge to the left side, tuck your right hand in and drag your left hand down the side of your body and out to the left. Shout the warrior's cry, "KI KI," as you lunge to the right and "So so" as you lunge left. You can increase your speed and then gradually slow down at the end of the exercise.

This exercise evokes the strength and confidence of the warrior in three ways. First, with our physical posture; our wide-legged stance grounds our lower body and connects us with the supportive energy of the earth, which increases our physical strength and gives us the confidence of having a stable foundation. Second, our movement is strong and openhearted, performed with a sense of fearlessness. Finally, we utter our warrior cry with delight and power. This strength, confidence, and brilliance is our windhorse. When our personal windhorse is supported, it is associated with good health and favorable conditions, both in terms of worldly activity and in terms of the spiritual path.

Three Mahamudra Exercises

The next three exercises are connected with particular aspects of meditation experience. In the Tibetan tradition, these experiences are mostly connected with what is called Mahamudra meditation.

Khenpo Rinpoche wrote this pithy verse that conveys the essence of instruction for Mahamudra meditation:

Look! Look at your own mind.
Look at its unborn ground.

Look at its unceasing play.
In this realm of luminosity-emptiness, relax.[2]

When you look directly at your own mind, you find there is no solid entity that can be called "mind." Trying to look at mind is like trying to grasp water with your fingers. There is something there, but it is indefinable. Mind is called the "unborn ground" because you never witness its birth, the first point when mind arises. We are told of our own physical birth, but we do not experience the birth of our own mind. If there is no arising of an entity, then there is no ceasing of it either. So mind neither arises nor ceases—it does not start, and it does not stop. But it is not a complete void, because from its unborn ground, the entire variety of our experiences manifest. This is mind's "unceasing play."

Thus mind is the union of emptiness and luminosity. Its quality of being an unborn ground expresses the emptiness of mind. The quality of mind's expression in unceasing play is its luminosity. When you see this, simply relax into that realm of luminosity-emptiness, just as it is. You do not need to apply any further technique.

It is best to work with Mahamudra once you have some extended practice in calm-abiding meditation as described previously. Whatever your meditation experience, you can apply the following instructions for specific techniques to work with the mind in these exercises. The first exercise connects with the meditative experience of nonthought, the second with clarity, and the third with bliss.

Shooting Arrow Yoga

When practicing the yoga of the shooting arrow,
Focus your eyes one-pointedly on your fingertip,
Rest in mind's nature, luminosity-emptiness.
Repeatedly meditate just like that,
And you will know mind's genuine abiding nature.[3]

Stand with your feet nearly one leg's length apart, and hold your hands with the index fingers pointing straight out and the other fingers curled into relaxed fists. Lunge toward the left, with your left leg bent and holding most of your weight, and your right leg straight. Your left foot should turn out in the same direction as your arms; your right foot should turn out to the right a little. Hold both arms outstretched to the left, which will necessitate some twisting of your upper body. Your right hip will turn in a little to facilitate the turn of your upper body, but do not move your hips completely to the left. Keep your body upright, not leaning in the direction of your arms (fig. 53).

Now draw your upper body back as if you are an archer pulling on a bow. Your left arm stays extended as your right arm bends completely so that the index finger comes level with your right shoulder. As you do this, bring the weight of your body back onto your right leg, which will bend, and straighten your left leg (fig. 54). Ensure that the knee of your right leg is pointing in the direction of your right foot, which now faces to the front at a right angle to

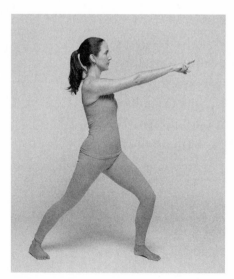
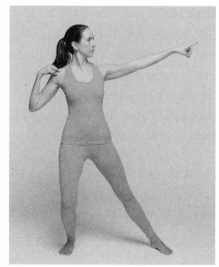

Figure 53

Figure 54

your left foot. Positioning your right leg at this angle sets it up for the next movement, in which you will follow your arm around to face the opposite direction.

Keep your gaze one-pointedly on your left index finger, but allow your gaze to be spacious so you do not strain your eyes. Begin to turn your upper body around to the right. Your feet will need to shuffle a little to keep your knee and foot aligned and to allow your body to complete a 180-degree turn. To aid this movement, try to encourage a sense of ease and relaxation in your hips. As you complete the turn, bring your right arm out to meet your left, so that both arms are held out to the right in front of you, as in the starting position, but now on the opposite side (fig. 55). Repeat the exercise by drawing your left arm back, keeping your right arm straight, and then turning around again to your left. You can keep flowing from one side to the other ten or twenty times (or as many times as you wish). Keep breathing naturally into your lower belly.

The movements in this exercise are precise. Keep your mind one-pointed. Rest your attention on the index finger of whichever arm

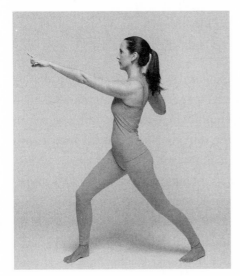

Figure 55

is extended, and when any distracting thoughts arise, simply notice them and bring your attention back to your fingertip. Sometimes, with this focus, there can be a tendency to hold your breath, so make sure you are still breathing into your lower belly.

The meditation experience that is emphasized through this exercise is that of nonthought. As you focus one-pointedly on your finger, allow whatever thoughts arise to simply fall away. You do not need to try to stop them from arising, for thoughts are the natural play of the mind, but do not follow them. Just as clouds pass through the sky, allow thoughts to gently pass through your mind, your realm of experience. When you do not interfere with thoughts—when you neither chase after them nor suppress them—they naturally liberate themselves.

Piercing Spear Yoga

> When practicing the yoga of the piercing spear,
> Gaze nakedly at your fingertips.
> Rouse clarity in your mind
> And rest in its space of luminosity-emptiness.
> Repeatedly meditate just like that,
> And let ordinary mind be laid bare.[4]

When first practicing this exercise, start by establishing the leg movements. Stand with your feet hip-width apart and parallel, then take one step forward with your left foot. Keep your hips square to the front. Now you are in the starting posture. Bend your knees, keep your torso upright, and allow your right heel to rise as you lower down. Go as far down as is comfortable for you. This movement requires strength in your legs and thighs, so gradually build up the depth to which you lower yourself. When you dip down, do not allow your knee to touch the floor—the lowest it should come is an inch or so above the floor. Then rise back up and lower your right heel to the ground.

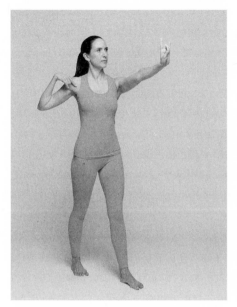

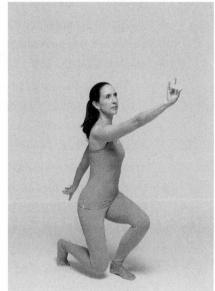

Figure 56   Figure 57

When you set up, step far enough forward on your left foot so that when you go down, your left knee does not extend over the toes of that foot. If you have any knee problems or injury, you need to be especially careful of honoring your own ability and working with that. You can do the exercise fully by just bending your knees very slightly and coming down only as far as feels workable. Repeat this motion ten or twenty times (or more). Then change legs and repeat on the opposite side the same number of times.

Once you are comfortable with the legs, add the hand and arm movements. Hold your hands in Threatening Mudra. When your left foot is forward, hold your left arm out in front and slightly upward with the wrist flexed while keeping your right hand level with your shoulder and your elbow drawn back and down. Look at the fingers of your left hand and also out into the space around them; keep your attention bright. As you bend your knees, simultaneously and energetically flick your left arm straight back and down and your right arm straight out in front, flexing your wrist; switch your gaze to the fingers of your right hand. Repeat a few times, then change to the other side (right leg and arm in front and the left back).

There is a sense of throwing a spear of attention and clarity out into space. The movement is powerful, but you hold the core of your body strongly so that the movement does not unbalance you. Make sure that your upper arms and shoulder muscles are strongly engaged and connected to your core body as you flick your arms out.

The meditation experience emphasized through this exercise is that of clarity—the brightness of the mind. As you flick your arm forward, focus on your fingers and the surrounding space with vibrant brightness. You get many opportunities to do this as your hands keep alternating. Do not try to hold on to the clarity as you change sides, simply flash on it and relax.

Swinging Swords Yoga

> When practicing the yoga of the swinging swords,
> Look inward and close the lower gate.
> Focus on physical sensations
> Relax in natural bliss-emptiness.
> Repeatedly meditate just like that,
> And bliss-emptiness, Mahamudra, will manifest.[5]

In this exercise, the leg movements are the same as in the previous exercise, Piercing Spear Yoga. Hold your hands with the palms flat and fingers together, like the smooth surface of a sword. Hold your palms toward each other with your elbows at the sides of your body. Your arms are going to make a circling motion, like a child playing at being a train, with one arm held higher than the other. Start with your left foot forward, your right arm held up, and your left arm lower. As you bend your knees, circle your arms in a smooth, continuous motion. Synchronize this movement with your legs so

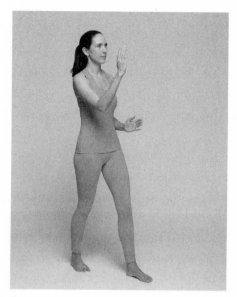 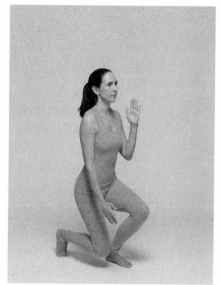

Figure 58   *Figure 59*

that when you return to standing, you will have completed one full revolution with your hands.

Keep your body upright throughout this exercise. For each cycle of the exercise—lowering down and raising back up again, one full rotation of the hands—gently close the lower gate at some point in the cycle. I prefer to do this as I bend down; you could start by doing that and then feel what works best for you. Once you have closed the lower gate, you do not need to keep it rigidly shut; simply close it, relax it, and allow any sensation that may arise to spread throughout your body. Train your gaze gently inward—meaning you do not look at anything externally, but your eyes are not closed either. Your gaze is just soft, and your focus of awareness is on the lower gate. Having practiced this a few times on one side, change to the other side. Over time, you will find that you can build up the number of repetitions you are able to do—from ten or twenty to fifty or sixty.

The meditation experience emphasized through this exercise is that of bliss—the feeling of softness and relaxation in your body. This is mainly done through working with the lower gate. You may find that pleasant sensations arise from closing the lower gate and that you can spread these throughout your body as you practice. You can also enhance this sensation by heightening the sensual quality of your movements, almost as if you were stroking a glorious cat with a glossy coat.

Bliss can be a difficult word for us to understand and experience, because we may have all sorts of expectations of how it *should* feel. Those expectations can get in the way of a direct experience of bliss. One of the important things to understand is that bliss is not an escapist experience of ecstasy in which suffering is no longer known or experienced. It is the sense of deep relaxation that comes when we no longer struggle with our present experience, no matter what the content of that experience is. Whether we grasp our experience tightly or reject it and try to push it away forcefully, we suffer. We become entangled in a dualistic struggle with that experience. If we can accept and truly be present to what is, we find something stable and sure at the core of all our experiences, an experience of spaciousness, openness, and relaxation.

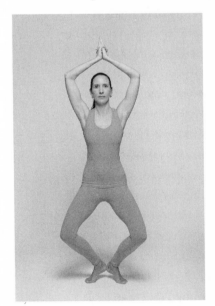

Figure 60

Indestructible Vajra Posture

A practice session traditionally concludes with this exercise. A *vajra*, or *dorjay* (*rdo rje*), is a Tibetan ritual implement shaped like one diamond atop another. First, stand with the heels of your feet together and your feet turned out. Rise up on the balls of your feet while still holding your heels together and lightly pressing into one another. (If you are able to hop straight up into this position, you can do so.) Bend your knees out to the sides so that they line up with the direction in which your feet are pointing—this creates the diamond shape in your lower body. Bring your hands together above the crown of your head; interlace your fingers apart from the middle fingers, which point straight up. If you can, bring the heels of your hands together. Bend your elbows out to the sides, creating the diamond shape in your upper body.

Start by holding this posture for as long as feels comfortable. Gradually increase the time as you become more familiar with it. You can hop out of this pose and then hop back into it, repeating it three, seven, or more times.

Keep breathing down into your lower belly as you hold this posture. Focus your eyes in front of you. Many people feel a lot of sensation in the body in this exercise; the thigh muscles, in particular, work hard to hold this pose. So your meditation can be simply to feel into the sensations that arise; rest your mind in awareness of bodily sensations.

Khenpo Rinpoche taught that this exercise is good preparation for the pain and discomfort we will experience at the time of death. When we die, most of us will likely have other plans for that day! Death comes unexpectedly even in old age and when we are sick. Many people struggle against the dying process. But if we can surrender to the experience when it comes, we will be able to engage it with more peace and equanimity.

This exercise gives us the opportunity to surrender to uncomfortable sensations and experience their essence directly. As we hold the posture, we can find a level of relaxation, even in the midst of discomfort. Not only will this help us at the time of death, but also with all experiences of physical pain. We train in looking at the essence of pain beyond all conceptual ideas about it or any storyline that we might apply to it.

However, it is important that we distinguish between the natural discomfort of holding a strenuous physical posture and the discomfort of holding the posture incorrectly or having a specific physical problem. In general, the discomfort inherent to the posture is felt in the muscles being used, while the discomfort of incorrect posture is felt in the joint areas. It is important to determine this for yourself and to check with a doctor if you have any concern.

If you feel pain in your knees, ensure that they are aligned with your feet. Try not to bend too low. You can start by just turning your knees out a little and gradually work on increasing the angle, being guided by the sensations in your knees and hips.

If your lower back does not feel comfortable, make sure you are not arching your lumbar spine and sticking your bottom out. Keep your pelvis aligned by dropping your tailbone down to the earth. Ensure that your back maintains its natural curves.

Closing Stretches

Here are some simple stretches to conclude your practice session that will ease you out of the session and help keep your body supple. If you would like to include other stretches, please do so.

Squat

The Squat (page 131) is a good stretch to hold for a few moments at the end of a session (fig. 61). Crouch down between your knees with

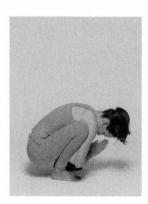

your hands between your legs on the floor. If you feel secure in this position, hold your hands together in prayer position with the outsides of your upper arms between your thighs. This position stretches out your lower back. If you feel comfortable and want to increase the stretch, press the insides of your thighs against your upper arms and push back on your legs with your upper arms. This will leverage your body forward. Hold this stretch for a few moments and focus on the sensations that arise in your body.

Figure 61

Forward Folds

From the previous position, place your hands on the floor, and release your head, neck, and shoulders forward so that they hang loosely. Gradually lift your buttocks up (fig. 62). You do not need to straighten your legs yet; allow your back to let go completely and flow downward. Release your head down toward the earth like a heavy weight. Allow any tension in your head, jaw, shoulders, and upper back to flow down into the earth. Surrender any rigidity to gravity. Imagine you are like a sheet hanging over a washing line that is positioned at the crease of your hips.

From this position, raise your buttocks higher until you feel a stretch in the backs of your thighs (fig. 63). You can raise up until your legs are straight if that feels workable. Otherwise, just keep lifting your buttocks upward and releasing your upper body down to the ground. Hold this position for a few moments. You can also slowly sway your body from side to side and see how this releases different areas of your hips and thighs. You can further release your muscles by breathing into any areas of intense sensation. Breath into the specific area, and on the exhalation, allow yourself to relax farther into the stretch.

While still hanging forward, bend one leg while straightening the other. Slowly alternate legs, while keeping your upper back and head loose and heavy (figs. 64 and 65). This allows the stretch

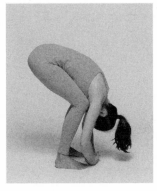
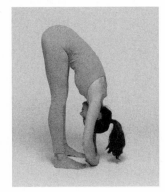

Figure 62   *Figure 63*

to get into different areas of your legs, hips, and back. You may want to hold the position a little where you find you are getting a good stretch.

Roll Spine to Standing

From this position, with both legs slightly bent (or more fully bent if you feel any strain in your lower back or the backs of your thighs), gradually roll your back upward to standing (fig. 66). Keep your upper body completely relaxed and heavy as you come up. Try to stack one vertebra on top of the next, starting at the bottom of your spine. At the end, bring your head upright and roll your shoulders back. Allow yourself to settle in standing position for a moment.

Stretch for the Front of the Thigh

From a simple standing position, take a big step forward with your left leg so your feet are about a full leg's length apart. Keep your body and both legs pointing forward. Bend your left leg deeply, bring your hands down to the floor, and drop your right knee to the floor. Untuck your toes so your shin can lie flat on the floor. You can also leave your toes tucked if that feels more stable for you. In either case, press into the floor with your foot: with untucked toes, press through the top of your foot and toes; with tucked toes, press

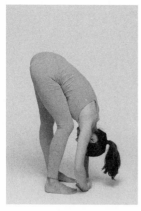

Figure 64

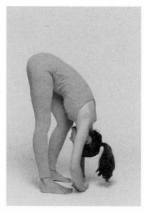

Figure 65

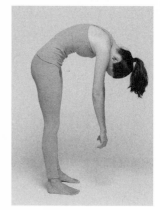

Figure 66

down through the ball of your foot
and spread your toes into the floor.
Make sure that your left knee does
not extend over the toes of that foot.
If your knee obscures your toes,
bring your left foot forward until
you can see them.

If you want to go further in this
stretch, bring your hands to your
left thigh, bringing your torso
upright (fig. 67). Wherever you are,

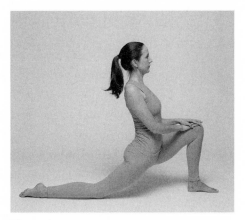

Figure 67

sink into your right thigh to deepen
the stretch. Keep squeezing your
left and right thighs toward each
other. Keep your tailbone dropping,
which will engage your abdominal
muscles. Then repeat the stretch on
the other leg.

Chest, Arms, and Shoulders

In simple standing position, interlace your fingers behind your back.
Draw your chest open. You can even
go into a little backbend with your

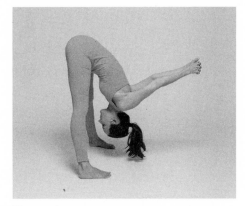

Figure 68

upper body. As you do this, drop your tailbone, as your bottom
may want to stick out in this posture. Keep your shoulders moving down, away from your ears. You can try clasping your hands
together strongly; the heels of your hands may even meet. Let your
heart open fully. Keep your head facing forward, floating comfortably at the top of your spine, with your chin slightly tucked.

To stretch farther, create more stability in your stance by widen-
ing your legs, then raise your arms up behind you and fold forward
over your legs. Let your clasped hands drop toward the floor behind
your head (fig. 68).

NATURAL ESSENCE DANCE

One of the best ways to loosen and release your body requires no formal technique at all. Just tune into the sensations in your body and follow the direction that it wants to move. Listen deeply to your body, and let go of conceptual mind and the movement it wants to impose on you. You may find it helpful to play soft music to bring out your body's natural movement. Use your meditation experience to tune into your bodily sensations, and follow the movement that your body needs in that moment. If possible, spend at least five minutes doing this at the end of the session.

BODY RUB

Once you have finished your session, take a moment to rub your body all over with flat palms. During this self-massage, appreciate your body and the work it has done; appreciate your ability to practice to whatever degree you are able; and be grateful you have this body-mind to practice with and this time and space for practice.

DEDICATION OF MERIT

Conclude the session with this dedication of merit, or one of your own choosing (for more on the dedication of merit, see page 24).

Milarepa's Aspiration Prayer
Sung at Rag-ma Jangchup Dzong

> May we live long and be free of illness,
> Enjoy freedom, great resources, and happiness.
> Next life, may we meet in the pure realm,
> May we always practice Dharma and benefit beings.[6]

Establishing a Regular Practice

It is good to practice lujong daily, but there is a lot of flexibility in terms of what that means. Some days, your session may last an hour; other days, it may last five minutes. It is fine to be realistic about working this practice into your schedule. Even a minute of lujong is extremely valuable if you really connect with the meditational aspect of the practice and move your body from that place. Initially, you will probably need to exert more effort to get to your practice session. However, over time, your body will naturally seek out these movement meditations and awareness practices.

It is not necessary to always practice the complete series of exercises. It is good to cycle through the complete series over a week or so and not habitually omit certain exercises, unless they are unsuitable for your body. Sometimes the exercises we simply dislike are the ones from which we will get the most benefit.

If you wish to perform the exercises in a different order to the one presented here, that is perfectly fine. You may structure some of your practice sessions based on what your body feels in the moment, so listen to how it wants to move and be guided by that.

The speed of the exercises can also vary. If you did not sleep well, or you overexerted yourself the day before, you may wish to practice more gently and do fewer repetitions. If you feel agitated or full of energy, you may feel that a vigorous session would be most beneficial. Practice the middle way: not pushing yourself too hard but also not holding back. Try to discover what is helpful to your body and work with that.

Good luck!

NOTES

INTRODUCTION

1. Throughout this book, each Tibetan term is transliterated in two different ways: the first gives an idea of how to say the word, while the second is the Wylie transliteration for those who read Tibetan.

2. Khenpo Tsültrim Gyamtso, conversation with the author, 2005.

CHAPTER 1. BUDDHIST YOGA

1. From Dharmakirti, *The Commentary on Valid Cognition* (Tib.: tshad ma rnam 'grel; Skt.: Pramana-varttika), quoted in Khenpo Tsültrim Gyamtso, *blo rtags kyi rnam gzhag rigs gzhung rgya mtsho'i snying po*, trans Ari Goldfield (New York: Nitartha International, 1997), 11.

2. Desire, anger, stupidity, jealousy, and arrogance.

3. Khenpo Tsültrim Gyamtso, letter, trans. Ari Goldfield.

4. These key points are what I have learned from my teachers (primarily the Tibetan masters Chögyam Trungpa Rinpoche and Khenpo Tsültrim Gyamtso Rinpoche) and their traditions of Tibetan Buddhist practice. There are certainly a wide variety of different explanations of these terms and topics within the panorama of Buddhist traditions, for just as doctors give different medicines to different patients, Buddhism traditionally presents and accommodates different explanations of its views and practices.

5. A founder of the Kagyü lineage of Tibetan Buddhism, Milarepa (1040–1123) is revered for having persevered through terrible hardship and austerity on his ultimately triumphant journey to enlightenment. His songs about his experiences and realization are renowned.

6. "Meeting with Paldarbum," trans. Willa Baker and Susan Skolnick (1997), from Tsang Nyon He-ru-ka, *rnal 'byor gyi dbang phyug chen*

po mi la ras pa'i rnam mgur [The Life and Songs of Milarepa, the Great Lord of the Yogis] (1488), retrieved from www.tibet.dk/pktc/ tibdtexts.php.

CHAPTER 2. RENUNCIATION
1. Unpublished, trans. Ari Goldfield.

CHAPTER 3. COMPASSIONATE BODHICHITTA
1. Shantideva, *The Way of the Bodhisattva*, trans. Padmakara Translation Group (Boston: Shambhala Publications, 1997), 34.
2. From the Tibetan text for the Karma Kagyu lineage preliminary (*ngondro*) practices, Dorje Wangchuk, *sgrub brgyud rin po che'i phreng ba karma kam tshang rtogs pa'i don brgyud las byung ba'i gsung dri ma med pa rnams bkod nas ngag 'don rgyun khyer gyi rim pa 'phags lam bgrod pa'i shing rta* [The Chariot for Traveling the Noble Path], trans. Ari Goldfield (unpublished), verse 9.
3. He-ru-ka, Tsang Nyon, *Rnal 'byor gyi dbang phyug chen po mi la ras pa'i rnam mgur* [The Life and Songs of Milarepa, the Great Lord of Yogis] (1488), retrieved from www.tibet.dk/pktc/tibdtexts.php, trans. Rose Taylor Goldfield, unpublished.
4. Chögyam Trungpa, *The Collected Works of Chögyam Trungpa* (Boston: Shambhala Publications, 2004), 3:398.
5. *Samadhi-raja-sutra* [The Buddha's Sutra Called "The King of Meditative States"], trans. Ari Goldfield, unpublished

CHAPTER 4. JOINING WITH NATURALNESS THROUGH THE PROFOUND VIEW OF TRUE REALITY
1. Orally quoted by Khenpo Tsültrim Gyamtso and translated by Ari Goldfield.
2. Tsang Nyon He-ru-ka, *rnal 'byor gyi dbang phyug chen po mi la ras pa'i rnam mgur* [The Life and Songs of Milarepa, the Great Lord of the Yogis] (1488), trans. Jim Scott, retrieved from www.tibet.dk/ pktc/tibdtexts.php.
3. Ibid., trans Jim Scott and Ari Goldfield.
4. Khenpo Tsültrim Gyamtso, unpublished verse, trans. Ari Goldfield.
5. For brevity's sake, the five stages in this presentation have been condensed into two. Books devoted to explaining all or some of these five stages in more detail include Khenpo Tsültrim Gyamtso,

Progressive Stages of Meditation on Emptiness (Oxford, UK: Long-chen Foundation, 1986); Khenpo Tsültrim Gyamtso, *The Sun of Wisdom* (Boston: Shambhala Publications, 2003); and Khenpo Tsül-trim Gyamtso, *Stars of Wisdom* (Boston: Shambhala Publications, 2010).

6. I recommend beginning with the books already listed for Khenpo Tsültrim Gyamtso and finding a teacher with whom you can have a direct relationship to help you in your study and practice. You can contact Ari Goldfield and myself through the Wisdom Sun website (www.wisdomsun.org), and you can also look on the Marpa Foundation website for other teachers' information (www.ktgrinpoche.org).

7. Kalu Rinpoche, unpublished poem (ca. 1980), in the possession of Susan Skolnick.

8. *bskyed rim gyi gsungs mgur* (Song of Meditating on the Generation Stage), trans. Ari Goldfield, from Tsang Nyon He-ru-ka, *rnal 'byor gyi dbang phyug chen po mi la ras pa'i rnam mgur* [The Life and Songs of Milarepa, the Great Lord of the Yogis] (1488), retrieved from www.tibet.dk/pktc/tibdtexts.php.

9. *gzer gsum gyi gsung mgur* (Song of the Three Nails), trans. Rose Taylor Goldfield, from Tsang Nyon He-ru-ka, *rnal 'byor gyi dbang phyug chen po mi la ras pa'i rnam mgur* [The Life and Songs of Milarepa, the Great Lord of the Yogis] (1488), retrieved from www. tibet.dk/pktc/tibdtexts.php.

10. Quoted in Wangchuk Dorje, *lhan cig skyes sbyor gyi zab khrid nges don rgya mtsho'i snying po phrin las 'od 'phro* [The Profound Instructions on Connate Union: The Radiant Activity at the Heart of an Ocean of Definitive Meaning], trans. Ari Goldfield, retrieved from www.dharmadownload.net/pages/english/Texts/texts_00 51.htm.

CHAPTER 7. HOW TO HOLD THE BODY

1. Dakpo Tashi Namgyal, "Illuminating the Natural State," trans. Ari Goldfield (unpublished manuscript).

CHAPTER 8. HOW TO HOLD THE MIND

1. Tsang Nyon He-ru-ka, *rnal 'byor gyi dbang phyug chen po mi la ras pa'i rnam mgur* [The Life and Songs of Milarepa, the Great Lord

of the Yogis] (1488), trans. Ari Goldfield, retrieved from www.tibet
.dk/pktc/tibdtexts.php.

2. Dakpo Tashi Namgyal, "Illuminating the Natural State," trans. Ari
Goldfield (unpublished manuscript).

3. David Gordon White, *The Alchemical Body* (Chicago: University
of Chicago Press, 1996), 46.

4. Dakpo Tashi Namgyal, "Illuminating the Natural State," trans. Ari
Goldfield (unpublished manuscript).

5. Tsang Nyon He-ru-ka, *rnal 'byor gyi dbang phyug chen po mi la
ras pa'i rnam mgur* [The Life and Songs of Milarepa, the Great Lord
of the Yogis] (1488), trans. Ari Goldfield, retrieved from www.tibet
.dk/pktc/tibdtexts.php.

CHAPTER 9. USING ADVERSITY TO ENHANCE THE PRACTICE OF BUDDHIST YOGA

1. Tsang Nyon He-ru-ka, *rnal 'byor gyi dbang phyug chen po mi la ras
pa'i rnam mgur* [The Life and Songs of Milarepa, the Great Lord of
the Yogis] (1488), trans. Ari Goldfield, retrieved from www.tibet.
dk/pktc/tibdtexts.php.

2. Chögyam Trungpa, unpublished manuscript.

3. A master of the Drukpa Kagyu lineage of Tibetan Buddhism who
lived from 1189 until 1258.

4. Jim Scott, trans., *The Eight Cases of Basic Goodness Not to Be
Shunned*, unpublished manuscript.

5. The head of the Karma Kagyu lineage of Tibetan Buddhism.

6. Wangchuk Dorje, *lhan cig skyes sbyor gyi zab khrid nges don rgya
mtsho'i snying po phrin las 'od 'phro* [The Profound Instructions
on Connate Union: The Radiant Activity at the Heart of an Ocean
of Definitive Meaning], trans. Ari Goldfield, retrieved from www
.dharmadownload.net/pages/english/Texts/texts_0051.htm.

7. Khenpo Tsültrim Gyamtso, talk delivered at Vajra Vidya Thrangu
House, Oxford, United Kingdom, 2000, trans. Ari Goldfield.

CHAPTER 10. PRACTICING WITH SYLLABLES AND SONG

1. For a complete commentary on this song and an overview of singing
as part of Buddhist practice, see Khenpo Tsültrim Gyamtso, *Stars
of Wisdom: Analytical Meditation, Songs of Yogic Joy, and Prayers*

of Aspiration, trans. Ari Goldfield and Rose Taylor Goldfield (Boston: Shambhala Publications, 2010). The melody to this song and others can be found at www.wisdomsun.org/index.php/downloads/articles-songs-and-more.

2. Tsang Nyon He-ru-ka, rnal 'byor gyi dbang phyug chen po mi la ras pa'i rnam mgur [The Life and Songs of Milarepa, the Great Lord of the Yogis] (1488), trans. Jim Scott, retrieved from www.tibet.dk/pktc/tibdtexts.php.

3. Khenpo Tsültrim Gyamtso, unpublished poems, trans. Rose Taylor Goldfield.

4. Such as that conducted by Dr. Michael Miller of the University of Maryland.

5. An epithet for Khenpo Tsültrim Gyamtso Rinpoche.

6. Khenpo Tsültrim Gyamtso, unpublished poems, trans. Ari Goldfield.

CHAPTER 11. PRACTICE IN DAILY LIFE

1. The "Song of Milarepa" is quoted in dpal sprul rin po che, kun bzang bla ma'i zhal lung (unpublished manuscript), 538. See also Patrul Rinpoche, The Words of My Perfect Teacher, trans. Padmakara Translation Group (Boston: Shambhala Publications, 1998).

2. "Samadhi refers to a state in which one is concentrated and not distracted. Paradoxically, it seems, the samadhi that sees everything to be like an illusion is the meditation one practices in the midst of all the distractions of thoughts and the objects that appear to the senses. When one remembers that all of these distractions are illusory, however, this constitutes the practice of this samadhi, and all the distractions are in fact friends of and enhancements to the meditation rather than hindrances or obstacles." From Khenpo Tsültrim Gyamtso, The Sun of Wisdom (Boston: Shambhala Publications, 2003), 53.

3. 'phags pa yang dag par sdud pa'i mdo [Compendium of Doctrine Sutra], quoted in Gampopa, lha rje bsod nams rin chen, dam chos yid bzhin gyi nor bu thar pa rin po che'i rgyan [Jewel Ornament of Liberation], (Kathmandu: Pema Karpo Translation Committee), 179. Electronic Tibetan pecha edition. Verse translated by Ari Goldfield.

4. Khenpo Tsültrim Gyamtso, unpublished poems, trans. Ari Goldfield.

5. Chögyam Trungpa, *The Collected Works of Chögyam Trungpa*, vol. 7 (Boston: Shambhala Publications, 2004).

CHAPTER 12. THE KEY POINTS OF BUDDHIST YOGIC EXERCISE

1. If you are familiar with tai chi or chi gong, the origin point is called *tan tien* in these traditions.

CHAPTER 13. EXERCISES

1. Khenpo Tsültrim Gyamtso, unpublished poems, trans. Ari Goldfield.

2. Khenpo Tsültrim Gyamtso, unpublished poems, trans. Rose Taylor Goldfield.

3. Khenpo Tsültrim Gyamtso, unpublished poems, trans. Rose Taylor Goldfield.

4. Khenpo Tsültrim Gyamtso, unpublished poems, trans. Rose Taylor Goldfield.

5. Khenpo Tsültrim Gyamtso, unpublished poems, trans. Ari Goldfield.

6. Tsang Nyon He-ru-ka, *rnal 'byor gyi dbang phyug chen po mi la ras pa'i rnam mgur* [The Life and Songs of Milarepa, the Great Lord of the Yogis] (1488), trans. Ari Goldfield, retrieved from www.tibet.dk/pktc/tibdtexts.php.

GLOSSARY

BODHICHITTA "The mind turned toward supreme enlightenment." Bodhichitta has two aspects: relative bodhichitta, arising from the cultivation of all-embracing love and compassion, is the vow to lead all sentient beings to the state of the complete and perfect enlightenment of buddhahood; ultimate bodhichitta is the true nature of reality itself. In Mahayana Buddhist practice, one cultivates and meditates on both types of bodhichitta.

BODHISATTVA "Courageous One of Enlightenment." A follower of the Mahayana path who cultivates the two types of bodhichitta. There are both ordinary bodhisattvas and noble bodhisattvas, the latter distinguished by their direct realization of the true nature of reality. Bodhisattvas are courageous because they take the vow to stay in samsara in order to benefit sentient beings, rather than seeking to escape from it. When bodhisattvas bring their wisdom and compassion to perfection, they become buddhas.

BUDDHA The teacher; an individual who has attained enlightenment by bringing wisdom that realizes the true nature of reality and compassion for all sentient beings to perfection. Shakyamuni, originally Prince Gautama, is the buddha of our era who gave the founding Buddhist teachings in this world; however, the Mahayana teaches that countless sentient beings have and will achieve buddhahood.

BUDDHA NATURE (Skt.: Sugata-garbha or Tathata-garbha) The true nature of mind—wisdom that is inherently pure and naturally endowed with the qualities of enlightenment. Thus, attaining enlightenment is not a matter of constructing something anew or acquiring something that one does not already possess; rather, it is about realizing one's own basic nature and potential.

DHARMA Defined as "something that holds its own essence," *dharma* refers to phenomena in general, and in particular to the phenomenon of Buddhist teachings. Buddhist teachings "hold" their practitioners back from falling into the confusion and suffering of samsara.

DHARMAKAYA One of the three kayas, or dimensions, of enlightenment (the other two are the *sambhogakaya* and *nirmanakaya*). The dharmakaya refers to the Buddha's enlightened mind, and the dharmakaya of natural purity refers to the true nature of that enlightened mind, which is also the true nature of the mind of every sentient being. In its nature, mind transcends conceptual fabrication; it is the essence of genuine reality. When one perfectly realizes the nature of mind, one attains the dharmakaya free of fleeting stains, awakening into the complete and perfect enlightenment of buddhahood. The sambhogakaya and the nirmanakaya are the two form kayas (*rupakaya*). The former appears to and teaches exclusively the noble bodhisattvas on the ten bodhisattva grounds; the latter appears to and teaches ordinary sentient beings and noble bodhisattvas alike.

EMPTINESS OF PHENOMENA The abiding reality of all phenomena, which is that they are empty of inherent nature, and ultimately empty of any conceptual notion of what they might be, even the notion of emptiness itself.

EQUALITY Contradictions, opposites, differences, and distinctions appear but do not truly exist. In genuine reality, opposites, differences, and distinctions are undifferentiable; they all have the same basic nature.

GENUINE REALITY Neither an object of the sense consciousnesses nor conceivable by thoughts, it is the true nature of all consciousnesses and their objects. It can be ascertained through analysis and experienced in meditation. When its experience becomes direct realization one becomes a noble bodhisattva; when this direct realization is perfected, one becomes a noble buddha.

GOTSANGPA (1189–1258) An emanation of Milarepa and a great early master of the Drukpa Kagyü lineage, four generations removed from Lord Gampopa, one of Milarepa's most accomplished disciples.

ILLUSION-LIKE SAMADHI *Samadhi* refers to a state in which one is concentrated and not distracted. Paradoxically, it seems, the illusion-like samadhi is the meditation one practices in the times between formal meditation sessions, in the midst of all the distractions of thoughts and the objects that appear to the senses. When one remembers that all of these distractions are illusory, this constitutes the practice of this samadhi, and all the distractions are in fact friends of and enhancements to the meditation rather than hindrances or obstacles.

KAGYÜ LINEAGE "The lineage of the teachings." One of the four major Tibetan Buddhist lineages (the others being Nyingma, Sakya, and Geluk), it originates with the Buddha Vajradhara (symbolizing the dharmakaya) to Tilopa, then Naropa, Marpa, Milarepa, and Gampopa. At that point, the lineage divides into many branches. The Karma Kagyü branch began with Gampopa's student Dusum Khyenpa, the first Karmapa. Today, Ogyen Trinley Dorje is the seventeenth Karmapa.

KARMA/KARMIC ACTIONS *Karma* literally means "action," but it can also refer to the results of actions as well. The actions that ordinary sentient beings take with body, speech, and mind, motivated by one or more kleshas and which result in suffering, are known as karmic actions.

KHENPO A title conferred upon a Tibetan Buddhist teacher that indicates mastery of scholarship.

KLESHAS The disturbing emotions and mental states that cause ordinary sentient beings suffering as a result of their not having realized the true nature of reality. The five main kleshas, also called the "five poisons," are: attachment or desire; aversion or anger; stupidity or mental dullness; pride; and jealousy.

LOWER GATE The lower gate is found at the bottom of the central channel that runs from the crown of the head down through the center of the body. The center of the lower gate is positioned between the pubic bone at the front and the coccyx bone at the base of spine. Closing the lower gate holds the subtle energies within the body and powers up the central channel.

MAHAMUDRA "Great Seal." A profound set of instructions that describe the true nature of reality as clarity-emptiness or bliss-emptiness, and how to meditate upon this true nature.

MAHAYANA The "Great Vehicle" of Buddhism: it is the path of the practice of the two types of bodhichitta; of wisdom and compassion together. Practitioners begin Mahayana practice by engendering love, compassion, and relative bodhichitta, and then training in the six transcendent practices (Skt.: paramitas): generosity, ethics, patience, diligence, concentration, and ultimate bodhichitta—the wisdom that realizes the true nature of reality—with the goal of attaining the enlightenment of the buddhas in order to lead all sentient beings to that same state.

MAITREYA The buddha of the future, the successor of Buddha Shakyamuni, traditionally depicted seated on a throne, Western-style. In the Mahayana schools of Buddhism, Maitreya is renowned for revealing five Dharma texts, *The Five Treatises of Maitreya*, to Asanga. Asanga was born in present-day Peshawar, in Pakistan, in the fourth century CE. He is said to be the half brother of Vasubandhu and together they are considered founders of the Yogachara school of Buddhism, as well as being major exponents of Abhidharma teachings.

MANJUSHRI The noble bodhisattva who is the embodiment of all the buddhas' wisdom. He is depicted wielding a flaming sword in his right hand, which represents transcendent wisdom cutting through ignorance and mistaken beliefs, such as duality. In his left hand he holds the Prajnaparamita sutra, representing the wisdom that realizes the emptiness of all phenomena.

MARPA THE TRANSLATOR (1012–1097) When Marpa was young, he had a ferocious temper and was known as a bully. His parents worried that he would either kill another or be killed himself, so they arranged for him to learn and practice the Dharma. Marpa made three arduous journeys to India and brought many teachings back with him to Tibet, which he translated into Tibetan in order to benefit the people of his native land. He became the teacher of Milarepa.

MILAREPA (1040–1123) A student of Marpa the Translator, this great yogi attained the state of buddhahood in a single lifetime and was one of the founders of the Kagyü lineage of Tibetan Buddhism. He is revered for having overcome suffering and having persevered through hardship and austerity in his triumphant journey to enlightenment. His songs about his experiences and realization are renowned.

NAROPA (11th century) A famous scholar at Nalanda University in India, Naropa left his academic post when he realized that although he was a master of the Dharma's words he had not fully inculcated their meaning. On the banks of a river, he met his teacher Tilopa, who was living as an outcaste, and endured the many difficult trials that Tilopa put him through before pointing out to him the true nature of his mind. At that point, Naropa realized the true meaning of Dharma and became a great siddha. He was the teacher of Marpa the Translator.

NIRVANA "Transcendence of suffering," the liberation from samsara that is achieved, according to the Shravaka-yana and Pratyeka-buddha-yana, when one realizes the selflessness of the individual sentient being. According to the Mahayana, the only authentic nirvana is the state of buddhahood, which, due to the perfection of the wisdom that realizes the emptiness of all phenomena, does not fall into the extreme of samsaric existence and, due to the perfection of compassion, does not fall into the extreme of peace (as the nirvana achieved by the shravaka and pratyeka-buddha arhats is thought to).

NOBLE TRUTHS The first teachings of the Buddha: (1) the truth of suffering; (2) the truth of the source of suffering; (3) the truth of the cessation of suffering; (4) the truth of the path to that cessation.

ORIGIN POINT The origin point is located just below the navel, deep in the center of the body and is important in many yogic traditions. As the center of our psychic and physical being and a potent place of connection between our different levels of being (the physical and subtle body, the conscious and subconscious mind) it is a source of great energy and insight.

PALTRUL RINPOCHE (1808–1887) A famous scholar and meditation master, and author of *Words of My Perfect Teacher*, a classic text on the stages of Buddhist practice, and *A Discourse Virtuous in the Beginning, Middle, and End*, a text that combines profound teachings on the view of genuine reality with meditation on Chenrezik, the bodhisattva who is the embodiment of compassion.

RENUNCIATION To abandon searching for happiness in the dualistic appearances of samsara.

RINPOCHE "Precious One." A title of highest esteem that Tibetan Buddhist students use to address their teacher.

SAMADHI Meditation; any meditative state of concentration. Literally defined as, "holding the mind one-pointedly on its object of focus."

SAMSARA The "cycle" of existence in which sentient beings who do not realize the true nature of reality wander from one lifetime to the next, experiencing constant suffering. More subtly, whenever one believes that oneself and the dualistic appearances of object and subject truly exist, one is vulnerable to the disturbing emotions and suffering, and so one is in samsara.

SELF-AWARENESS Non-dual, inexpressible awareness that both the Mind-Only and Empty-of-Other schools assert is the true nature of mind. The Mind-Only school asserts self-awareness to be a truly existent entity;

whereas the Empty-of-Other school asserts that self-awareness is not a truly existent entity, it is luminosity-emptiness inseparable.

SELFLESSNESS OF THE INDIVIDUAL When sentient beings believe the self—the object referred to by thoughts of "I" and "me"—to be truly existent, that is a confused belief that is the source of all suffering. However, in genuine reality, the self does not exist. Therefore, the "I" and "me" that appear in relative reality are dependently arisen mere appearances. This view of selflessness is held in common by all Buddhist philosophical schools.

SELF-LIBERATION Primarily, the freedom that is an inherent quality of the true nature of appearances and mind. Since appearances are by nature appearance-emptiness, and thoughts and emotions are by nature clarity-emptiness, they need no outside liberator to set them free. Like when one is bound by iron chains in a dream the perfect remedy is to realize that one is dreaming, one must only realize the true nature of one's experiences to gain liberation from whatever difficulties they may present.

In the Mahamudra and Dzogchen traditions, phenomena are described as self-liberated because they are "self-arisen," meaning that they have no truly existent causes for their arising.

SHAMATHA "Calm-abiding" meditation. When mind's distracted movements *calm* down, and mind *abides* one-pointedly on the meditation's object of focus.

SHANTIDEVA (7th–8th centuries) Great Indian master and author of *Entering the Bodhisattvas' Way*, a famous compendium of Mahayana view and practice.

SIDDHA "One who has gained accomplishment." A practitioner who has realized the true nature of reality.

TILOPA (10th–11th centuries) A great Indian master who abandoned life as a prince to seek realization on the path of Dharma. However, he did not gain realization until he learned how to meditate while working at ordinary jobs—crushing sesame seeds by day, and as a caller and janitor at a beerhouse by night. He became the main teacher of Naropa.

TRULKHOR is the term for physical yogic exercise that is taught in the Vajrayana and that has many specific movements to learn.

VAJRAYANA "Adamantine vehicle." It is the set of Mahayana practices that one learns in stages under the supervision of a qualified teacher, and which practitioners keep secret from those who have not been initiated into the same levels of practice.

YOGA "To join with naturalness." Any practice that helps its practitioners to realize the true nature of reality.

YOGI/YOGINI Male (yogi) and female (yogini) practitioners who have "arrived at naturalness," meaning that they have realized the true nature of reality to one degree or another. Thus, there are shravaka-yogis, pratyekabuddha-yogis, bodhisattva-yogis, and buddha-yogis, the last of these being the greatest yogis of all.

RESOURCES

For information on events, teaching sessions, audio recordings, community news, and song recordings, please visit www.wisdomsun.org. To join our e-mail list, please contact us at info@wisdomsun.org.

RECOMMENDED READING

Freeman, Richard. *The Mirror of Yoga: Awakening the Intelligence of Body and Mind* (Boston, MA: Shambhala Publications, 2012).

Gyamtso, Khenpo Tsültrim. *Stars of Wisdom* (Boston, MA: Shambhala Publications, 2010).

———. *The Sun of Wisdom* (Boston, MA: Shambhala Publications, 2003).

Stone, Michael. *Freeing the Body, Freeing the Mind: Writings on the Connections between Yoga and Buddhism* (Boston, MA: Shambhala Publications, 2010).

INDEX